# Psychological Approaches to Generalized Anxiety Disorder

---

---

# Psychological Approaches to Generalized Anxiety Disorder

## A Clinician's Guide to Assessment and Treatment

Holly Hazlett-Stevens, Ph.D.
University of Nevada, Reno

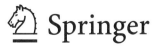 Springer

Holly Hazlett-Stevens, Ph.D.
University of Nevada, Reno
Department of Psychology/298
Reno, NV 89557
USA
hhazlett@unr.edu

ISBN: 978-0-387-76869-4        e-ISBN: 978-0-387-76870-0
DOI: 10.1007/978-0-387-76870-0

Library of Congress Control Number: 2008928768

Printed on acid-free paper

9 8 7 6 5 4 3 2 1

springer.com

*To Chris and Jack*

# Acknowledgments

The ideas and clinical practices contained in this book are based on the innovative work of many researchers and colleagues in the field. I have had the great fortune of working with two exceptional mentors, Tom Borkovec and Michelle Craske, both of whom have influenced my thinking on this topic immeasurably. This book certainly would not have been possible without their teachings and support throughout my career, not to mention their brilliant contributions to our field. The cognitive-behavioral therapy techniques described in this book are based largely on the work of Tom Borkovec, who has been developing and refining GAD treatment approaches for most of his career. In collaboration with Douglas Bernstein, he developed a systematic progressive relaxation method widely recognized for its effectiveness. His more recent work with colleagues Louis Castonguay and Michelle Newman led to the integration of interpersonal and experiential therapy approaches. I consider myself incredibly fortunate to have worked with this group at Penn State, and I am greatly indebted to Tom and his collaborators as well as to Michelle Craske and the many other psychologists involved in my training over the years. My thinking also continues to be enhanced by the bright and creative graduate students in my laboratory: Michael Ritter, Amanda Drews, Deacon Shoenberger, Stephanie Spear, Larry Pruitt, Angie Collins, Kirsten Lowry, and Susan Daflos.

I would also like to thank Martin Antony for inviting me to write this book for his anxiety series as well as Sharon Panulla and Jennifer Hadley at Springer for all of their assistance in the preparation of this manuscript. Finally, a special thanks to Larry Pruitt for his essential contributions to the second chapter and to Susan Daflos for all of her wonderful help preparing the final manuscript for production.

# About the Author

Holly Hazlett-Stevens received her Ph.D. in clinical psychology from the Pennsylvania State University in 1999. Under the mentorship of Dr. Thomas Borkovec, she studied the nature of anxiety and worry as well as cognitive behavioral therapy for generalized anxiety disorder (GAD). From 1999–2001, Dr. Hazlett-Stevens was a post-doctoral fellow in the Department of Psychology at the University of California, Los Angeles under the mentorship of Dr. Michelle Craske. There she received training in cognitive behavioral treatment for panic disorder, coordinated panic disorder intervention research projects, and continued her own program of anxiety and worry research.

In 2002, Dr. Hazlett-Stevens joined the faculty of the Psychology Department at the University of Nevada, Reno, where she is currently an Associate Professor. She has conducted psychological research in the areas of worry, anxiety disorders, and relaxation for the past 10 years, resulting in the publication of over 20 articles and book chapters. She also co-authored *New Directions in Progressive Relaxation Training* with Douglas A. Bernstein and Thomas D. Borkovec. Her self-help book, *Women Who Worry Too Much: How to Stop Worry & Anxiety from Ruining Relationships, Work, & Fun* was released by New Harbinger publications in 2005. Dr. Hazlett-Stevens has served as an ad-hoc reviewer for several academic and professional journals in the area of clinical psychology, and she has been listed in several Who's Who lists.

# Contents

# Chapter 1
# Diagnosis, Clinical Features, and Theoretical Perspectives

Generalized anxiety disorder (GAD) is a chronic anxiety condition characterized by excessive and uncontrollable worry and associated somatic symptoms. Unlike other anxiety disorders, GAD involves diffuse anxiety in the absence of a specific feared object, class of stimuli, or situation. Individuals suffering from GAD instead fear and avoid an array of subtle internal and external stimuli. Worry, a cognitive process in which individuals anticipate threatening outcomes and events, becomes a strategy to detect and to cope with impending threat. As a result, these individuals live in a constant state of hypervigilance. Because anticipated threats typically are highly unlikely or vague in nature, the innate human capability to plan ahead by thinking into the future generates subjective anxiety and tension rather than constructive problem-solving action. Chronic muscle tension, sleep disturbance, and a variety of other symptoms also develop. Individuals with this anxiety condition often suffer from some degree of functional impairment, ranging from trouble concentrating at work to strained interpersonal relationships. Severe subjective distress and persistent concern about excessive worry and chronic anxiety symptoms are common as well.

While GAD is characterized by chronic and diffuse anxiety without a clear target, some degree of worry, general anxiety symptoms, and associated neurobiological factors can be found across the other anxiety disorders. For this reason, Barlow (1988) famously proposed that GAD may be the "basic" anxiety disorder. That is, the basic processes underlying GAD may underlie the other anxiety disorders as well. Thus, the more we learn about the development and maintenance of GAD, the better we may understand how other anxiety disorders develop and persist. Indeed, GAD first appeared in the *Diagnostic and Statistical Manual of Mental Disorders* (DSM) diagnostic system as a residual diagnostic category, assigned only when no other anxiety disorder diagnosis could be made. In 1987, the American Psychiatric Association acknowledged GAD as a separate diagnostic entity; they further refined GAD diagnostic criteria in 1994. In accord with these developments in the diagnostic system, epidemiological information has become increasingly available. This chapter briefly reviews the history of GAD diagnosis and presents the current diagnostic definition provided by the American Psychiatric Association. Essential findings from epidemiological research are discussed as well. Finally, current theoretical approaches explaining how GAD develops and maintains over time are presented.

H. Hazlett-Stevens, *Psychological Approaches to Generalized Anxiety Disorder*,
doi: 10.1007/978-0-387-76870-0, © Springer Science+Business Media, LLC 2008

## Generalized Anxiety Disorder Diagnosis

The diagnosis "generalized anxiety disorder" began with the third edition of the DSM (DSM-III; American Psychiatric Association 1980), but was included only as a residual diagnosis. Seven years later, GAD was recognized as an independent diagnosis that could be made even when other anxiety disorder diagnoses were present (DSM-III-R; American Psychiatric Association 1987). GAD diagnostic criteria were updated in several ways during the latest DSM revision (DSM-IV; American Psychiatric Association 1994). This revised current GAD diagnostic definition contains somatic symptoms most often associated with worry and anxious apprehension rather than the physiological hyperarousal symptoms associated with many other anxiety disorders.

### *History of GAD Diagnosis*

Chronic anxious disturbance first appeared in the DSM as an "anxiety reaction" (DSM-I; American Psychiatric Association 1952). The revised term "anxiety neurosis," was a broad diagnostic category for excessive and chronic anxiety without behavioral avoidance of circumscribed external objects or situations (DSM-II; American Psychiatric Association 1968). The diagnostic label of GAD was first available in 1980, with the third edition of the DSM (DSM-III; American Psychiatric Association 1980). Two new diagnostic categories replaced the previous category of anxiety neurosis: panic disorder and GAD. Diagnosis of GAD required symptoms such as anxious apprehension, worry or rumination, tension, restlessness, physiological anxious arousal, and hypervigilance, persisting for at least 1 month (Mennin, Heimberg, & Turk 2004). However, GAD diagnosis was only possible if the individual failed to meet diagnostic criteria for any of the other DSM-III anxiety disorders during that time period.

When the DSM was again revised (DSM-III-R; American Psychiatric Association 1987), GAD became a separate diagnostic category rather than a residual one. In the DSM-III-R, GAD was diagnosed when an individual reported excessive or unrealistic worry about at least two life domains and the worry was accompanied by at least six anxiety symptoms from a list of eighteen. This symptom list contained a diverse array of somatic symptoms, such as physical muscle tension, and cognitive symptoms, such as hypervigilance. Most symptoms reflected autonomic nervous system arousal, such as accelerated heart rate and shortness of breath. GAD symptoms were required for at least 6 months, replacing the previous 1-month DSM-III criterion. A GAD diagnosis could be made if another diagnosis was present, assuming that the anxiety and worry supporting the GAD diagnosis was unrelated to that additional disorder. Although these revisions likely reduced diagnostic confusion at that time, many of the particular criteria selected for GAD diagnosis were not supported by subsequent research. For example, unrealistic worry was not proving to be a useful distinction. Abel and Borkovec (1995) found that individuals with GAD and nonanxious control group individuals reported that their worry was unrealistic to equivalent degrees. In contrast, reports of "uncontrollable" worry—worry experienced as difficult to control—did discriminate individuals with GAD from nonanxious control individuals (Craske, Rapee, Jackel, & Barlow 1989). Furthermore, many of the eighteen possible somatic symptoms did not reflect the physiology and phenomenology of GAD accurately. Symptoms of autonomic nervous system hyperarousal were not frequently endorsed by GAD individuals (Marten, Brown, Barlow, Borkovec, et al. 1993). When physiology was measured directly in laboratory studies, evidence of elevated autonomic nervous system arousal was not observed (e.g., Hoehn-Saric, McLeod, & Zimmerli 1989). Instead, GAD physiology was characterized by reduced autonomic variability (Lyonfields, Borkovec, & Thayer 1995; Thayer, Friedman, & Borkovec 1996) and increased muscle tension (Hoehn-Saric et al. 1989; Hazlett, McLeod, & Hoehn-Saric 1994).

## *Current GAD Diagnostic Definition*

GAD diagnostic criteria were revised most recently in 1994 (DSM-IV; American Psychiatric Association 1994). Consistent with the research findings just described, the term "unrealistic" was eliminated and replaced with the requirement that worry be perceived as uncontrollable. Clinicians no longer needed to establish that worry about two or more life spheres was present. Instead, the worry must be considered excessive and span across different life activities. Finally, the list of associated symptoms required for diagnosis changed substantially. Autonomic hyperarousal symptoms were dropped, and the remaining symptoms were re-arranged into a list of six. Diagnosis now requires at least three of six anxiety symptoms, consisting of restlessness, fatigue, difficulty concentrating, irritability, muscle tension, and sleep disturbance. The requirement that symptoms persist for at least 6 months was retained in the DSM-IV. As with other diagnoses, symptoms should not be due to the direct physiological effects of a substance or general medical condition, and clients must experience clinically significant distress or functional impairment. GAD remains a separate diagnostic category, but the anxiety and worry should not be limited to features of another Axis I disorder. The American Psychiatric Association recently updated the text accompanying previously published DSM-IV criteria (DSM-IV-Text Revision; American Psychiatric Association 2000) without revising actual diagnostic criteria. See Chap. 3 for a discussion of differential diagnosis considerations and diagnostic assessment procedures.

The current DSM-IV diagnostic criteria for GAD are largely compatible with the current international diagnostic criteria established by the World Health Organization (WHO), the *International Classification of Diseases and Related Health Problems, 10th edition* (ICD-10; WHO 1992). Nevertheless, some notable differences can be found. The ICD-10 does not require the worry to be excessive and uncontrollable, nor does it require that the worry and anxiety cause significant clinical distress or impairment. Associated somatic symptoms required for diagnosis contain many of the autonomic hyperactivity symptoms that were dropped from the DSM during its latest revision. In contrast to the DSM-IV, GAD cannot be diagnosed with the ICD-10 when major depressive disorder or selected other anxiety disorders are present. Although an acceptable degree of reliability between diagnostic measures based on DSM-IV and ICD-10 criteria have been reported (Starcevic & Bogojevic 1999), only half a sample of individuals meeting ICD-10 criteria for GAD also received a GAD diagnosis when DSM-IV criteria were applied (Slade & Andrews 2001). Ruscio, Lane, Roy-Byrne, Stang, et al. (2005) examined the specific impact of the DSM-IV excessive worry criterion. Once this particular diagnostic criterion was eliminated, the estimated lifetime prevalence of GAD increased by approximately 40%. Taken together, these research findings suggest that more cases of GAD can be identified with the ICD-10 while the DSM-IV diagnostic criteria appear more stringent. The DSM-IV system receives more widespread use than the ICD-10 for diagnosis of GAD.

## Epidemiology and Related Statistics

Estimates of GAD prevalence were first obtained with DSM-III diagnostic criteria, and later large-scale epidemiological research employed DSM-III-R criteria. The most recent investigation of GAD prevalence using the current DSM-IV diagnostic criteria reported a lifetime prevalence rate estimate of 5.7% (Kessler, Berglund, Demler, Jin, et al. 2005) and a 1-year prevalence rate estimate of 3.1% (Kessler, Chiu, Demler, & Walters 2005). GAD is more often diagnosed in women compared to men, although this gender distribution has not always been replicated in research conducted outside the United States. GAD is typically associated with an early age of onset, but this chronic condition may be common among older adults as well. Common additional diagnoses include social anxiety disorder and the depressive disorders. Individuals with GAD often seek help from medical practitioners, wanting relief from anxiety-related somatic complaints as well as comorbid medical conditions.

### *Prevalence and Course*

United States population estimates of GAD prevalence were first obtained from the Epidemiological Catchment Area (ECA) study with DSM-III diagnostic criteria. The 1-year prevalence of GAD was then estimated at 3.8% (Blazer, Hughes, George, Swartz, & Boyer 1991). A later project named the National Comorbidity Survey (NCS) interviewed a sample of more than 8000 American adults. Using DSM-III-R criteria, an estimated current prevalence of 1.6%, an estimated 1-year prevalence of 3.1%, and a lifetime prevalence rate of 5.1% were reported for GAD (Kessler, McGonagle, Zhao, Nelson, et al. 1994; Wittchen, Zhao, Kessler, & Eaton 1994). The NCS recently was replicated with a larger sample (9282 respondents) using the current DSM-IV diagnostic criteria. Despite notable changes in GAD diagnostic criteria, the 1-year estimated prevalence rate was 3.1% (Kessler, Chiu, et al. 2005), the same rate obtained by the original NCS study. The lifetime prevalence rate was estimated at 5.7% (Kessler, Berglund, et al. 2005), slightly higher than the earlier 5.1% estimate.

Epidemiological investigations outside the U.S. tend to yield similar results. One study (Faravelli, Degl'Innocenti, & Giardinelli 1989) assessed 1110 Italian citizens believed to represent the general population of Florence, Italy. A current GAD prevalence estimate of 2.8% and a lifetime GAD prevalence estimate of 5.4% were reported, based on DSM-III-R diagnostic criteria. A community survey conducted in rural South Africa using DSM-IV criteria estimated current GAD prevalence at 3.7% (Bhagwanjee, Parekh, Paruk, Petersen, & Subedar 1998). The Netherlands Mental Health Survey and Incidence Study (NEMESIS; Bijl, Ravelli, & van Zessen 1998) involved in-person diagnostic interviews from over 7000 respondents. Lifetime and 1-year prevalence rates for GAD, as defined by DSM-III-R diagnostic criteria, were 2.3% and 1.2% respectively. A comparable 1-year GAD prevalence estimate of 1.1% was obtained in Ontario, Canada, also based on DSM-III-R criteria (Offord, Boyle, Campbell, Goering, et al. 1996). Thus, estimates of GAD prevalence for Dutch and Canadian populations were a bit lower than the rates reported in U.S. epidemiological studies. However, one final investigation using DSM-IV diagnostic criteria found a much lower 1-year GAD prevalence rate of only 0.4% in a Mexican urban sample (Medina-Mora, Borges, Lara, Benjet, et al. 2005). According to the authors, many of the prevalence rates found in this investigation were lower than those obtained in other countries possibly because of differences in Mexican culture. Factors such as greater perceived social support associated with "familism" may protect Mexican individuals from many of the mental disorders studied. These authors also acknowledged that differences in prevalence rates could be due to methodological limitations. For example, the reliability and validity of the survey version used in this investigation had not been established in Mexico.

The course of GAD is typically quite chronic. One large-scale investigation, the Harvard/Brown Anxiety Research Program (HARP) studied the natural course of anxiety disorders with a prospective longitudinal design (Yonkers, Warshaw, Massion, & Keller 1996). Patients recruited from various psychiatric and medical settings were followed for 5 years with periodic repeated assessments of their symptoms. Of the patients who received an initial diagnosis of GAD at their first assessment, only 15% experienced a period of remission within the first year and only 25% experienced a period of remission within the first 2 years (Yonkers et al. 1996). This figure rose only to 38% by the end of the 5-year study period (Yonkers, Dyck, Warshaw, & Keller 2000). GAD has been associated with significant functional impairment (Wittchen et al. 1994) as well as low life satisfaction and poor perceived well-being (Stein & Heimberg 2004).

## Demographic Features

Women in the U.S. are twice as likely as men to suffer from GAD, both among the general population (Wittchen et al. 1994) and among clinical treatment-seeking samples (Woodman, Noyes, Black, Schlosser, & Yagla 1999). A similar degree of female pre-dominance was found in the investigations conducted in the Netherlands (Bijl et al. 1998) and in Canada (Offord et al. 1996). However, this gender distribution may be culturally specific. The epidemiological survey conducted in South Africa revealed that rates of GAD were significantly higher in men than women (Bhagwanjee et al. 1998).

Many experts associate GAD with an early age of onset. Indeed, many clients report they have been worriers all their lives or that their worry became excessive during the transition from adolescence to adulthood. Empirical support for such clinical observations was provided by Hoehn-Saric, Hazlett, and McLeod (1993). Age of onset was examined among 103 adults seeking treatment for GAD. The majority (64%) reported an onset of symptoms before age 20, whereas age of onset sometime after the age of 20 characterized the remaining participants. Among the early-onset group, symptoms began by age 10 for 15% of these participants and between ages 10 and 19 years for the remaining 85%. For the later-onset group, symptoms most often began during the twenties (ages 20–29), accounting for 43% of these participants. Symptom onset between ages 30 and 39 were reported by 31% of these participants, and 22% reported symptom onset after age 40. Thus, GAD symptoms typically appear for the first time during childhood, adolescence, and early adulthood. Compared to the participants reporting adult-onset GAD, individuals reporting GAD onset in childhood or adolescence appeared to have experienced more childhood difficulties. The early-onset group also scored higher than the adult-onset group on self-report measures of various anxiety-related traits and current interpersonal difficulties.

GAD may be common later in the lifespan as well. The original NCS epidemio-logical study found that GAD was most common among adults who were 45 years old or older and least common among respondents in the 15–24 year-old age group (Wittchen et al. 1994). Similar results were obtained in the NCS replication study, in which the highest prevalence rate for GAD was found among individuals age 45–59 (Kessler, Berglund, et al. 2005). Increasing interest in the nature, assessment, and treatment of GAD among older adults—age 60 years or older—has developed over the past 15 years. In their review of this literature, Beck and Averill (2004) suggested that current DSM diagnostic criteria may not capture notable anxiety symptoms among the elderly. The considerable overlap between GAD and major depressive episode diagnostic criteria may be especially problematic for the assessment of older adults, as these individuals tend to describe their symptoms as somatic complaints rather than as cognitive or emotional problems. Nevertheless, GAD among elderly individuals is associated with elevated anxiety, worry, depression, and social fears, none of which are simply explained by the normal aging process (Beck, Stanley, & Zebb 1996). Despite epidemiological findings of high GAD prevalence among younger Americans, Beck and Averill argued that the high prevalence of GAD found within nursing home settings warrants further attention. Reported GAD prevalence rates range from 3.5% to 6% among nursing home residents, typically over 75 years of age (Junginger, Phelan, Cherry, & Levy 1993; Parmelee, Katz, & Lawton 1993).

## Comorbid Conditions

Most individuals suffering from GAD meet diagnostic criteria for other DSM diagnoses as well (e.g., Sanderson & Barlow 1990). Social anxiety disorder is considered the most common additional anxiety disorder diagnosis, as 59% of individuals with GAD also suffer from social anxiety disorder (Sanderson, DiNardo, Rapee, & Barlow 1990). In regards to comorbid depressive disorders, 42% of individuals diagnosed with GAD reported a history of major depressive episodes (Brawman-Mintzer, Lydiard, Emmanuel, Payeur, et al. 1993). Among treatment-seeking individuals diagnosed with dysthymia, over 65% also were diagnosed with GAD (Pini, Cassano, Simonini, Savino, et al. 1997). Individuals with GAD may present with personality disorder features as well, particularly those within Cluster C, the "anxious/fearful" cluster. Sanderson and colleagues found that almost half (49%) of their GAD clinical sample were diagnosed with a comorbid Axis II disorder (Sanderson, Wetzler, Beck, & Betz 1994). Among these Axis II conditions, avoidant and dependent personality disorders were diagnosed most often (Sanderson & Wetzler 1991). In the later study (Sanderson et al. 1994), these authors further found a specific link between GAD and obsessive-compulsive personality disorder (OCPD). The association observed between GAD and OCPD was second only to the association found between social phobia and avoidant personality disorder.

Individuals with GAD often visit general medical practitioners, such as primary care physicians. Roy-Byrne and Wagner (2004) reviewed published GAD prevalence rates within the primary care setting. They found that 2.8% to 8.5% of medical patients visiting their physician for any reason also were suffering from GAD, approximately twice the rate reported in community epidemiological surveys. Many individuals with GAD first seek treatment for their anxiety-related symptoms in medical settings, wanting relief from insomnia, restlessness, or chronic muscle tension. In addition, GAD may co-occur with medical conditions, particularly those involving the gastrointestinal system. Gastrointestinal problems such as ulcers and stomach distress appear to accompany GAD more than other medical conditions (Sareen, Cox, Clara, & Asmundson 2005). Additional investigations have examined the link between GAD and irritable bowel syndrome (IBS). Approximately 37% of a clinical GAD sample also met diagnostic criteria for IBS (Tollefson, Tollefson, Pederson, Luxenberg, & Dunsmore 1991), and 34% of an IBS patient sample had a lifetime history of GAD (Lydiard 1992). We since found a high degree of comorbidity between GAD and IBS among a general college student sample (Hazlett-Stevens, Craske, Mayer, Chang, & Naliboff 2003; Drews & Hazlett-Stevens, in press). Not surprisingly, GAD diagnosis is associated with high utilization of medical services (Roy-Byrne & Wagner 2004).

# Current Theoretical Approaches

Several biological and psychological influences may contribute to the development and/or maintenance of GAD. Neurobiological theories (e.g., Sinha, Mohlman, & Gorman 2004) have implicated neuroanatomical structures including the amygdala and hippocampus as well as neurochemical systems such as gamma-aminobutyric acid (GABA), norepinephrine (NE), and serotonin (5-HT). The neuropeptide chole-cystokinin (CCK) and the limbic-hypothalamic-pituitary-adrenal axis (LHPA axis) have been linked to normal anxiety and stress responses as well as to pathological anxiety. Additionally, a variety of cognitive and cognitive-behavioral models of GAD have appeared in the academic literature over the past couple of decades. Information-processing theory (e.g., MacLeod & Rutherford 2004) highlights the importance of automatic cognitive processes that are biased toward the detection and interpretation of threat. From this perspective, cognitive tendencies to selectively attend to threatening stimuli and to interpret ambiguous information as threatening play a causal role in the development of GAD symptoms. In his meta-cognitive account of GAD, Wells (2004) proposed that worry first develops as a way to cope with anticipated threat, naturally leading to meta-cognitive beliefs about the benefits of worry. However, GAD may develop when negative beliefs about worry also are activated. According to this view, threatening appraisals of worry and further worry about worry itself lead to counterproductive behavior and attempts to suppress or control worrisome thoughts. As a result, the belief that worry and anxiety are dangerous only escalates subjective distress and perpetuates anxious disturbance. A final theoretical model implicates a construct known as "intolerance of uncertainty" in the etiology and maintenance of GAD (Dugas, Buhr, & Ladouceur 2004). That is, a tendency to experience negative cognitive, behavioral, and emotional reactions to uncertain events causes elevated distress and impaired functioning in a variety of everyday ambiguous situations. GAD therefore develops from chronic maladaptive beliefs that uncertainty itself is threatening and must be avoided. All of these theories are presented in greater depth in an excellent text entitled *Generalized anxiety disorder: Advances in research and practice*, edited by R.G. Heimberg, C.L. Turk, and D.S. Mennin (2004).

The cognitive-behavioral treatment described in this book was based largely on two prominent theoretical perspectives: the integrative etiological model of GAD developed by Barlow and colleagues and the avoidance theory of worry and GAD proposed by Borkovec and colleagues. This latter theoretical model was recently expanded by Mennin and colleagues to incorporate possible emotional regulation deficits. Both theoretical approaches are reviewed here and are summarized for clients during early psychoeducation treatment sessions.

## *An Integrative Theoretical Model of GAD*

Barlow (1988) originally proposed that all anxiety disorders, including GAD, stem from a synergy of general biological vulnerabilities, such as neurobiological and genetic factors, and general psychological vulnerabilities, such as early experiences characterized by unpredictability or a lack of control over one's environment. These vulnerabilities do not appear specific to GAD. Rather, they reflect general tendencies toward negative affect and threat perception that can lead to various manifestations of emotional disturbance. In a recently updated version of this model, Roemer, Orsillo, and Barlow (2002) began with this basic propensity to react to situations with anxiety, other negative emotions, and heightened physiological arousal. This general tendency, sometimes referred to as "negative affectivity" or "neuroticism," is only considered a diathesis, leaving a person vulnerable to emotional disorders if significant stressful life events later occur. The tendency to experience heightened anxious arousal interacts with stressful event(s), thereby producing intense levels of anxiety. As biological and psychological vulnerabilities interact with stressful life events, a state of anxious apprehension involving increased tension and hypervigilance to threat result. The individual soon learns to perceive threat easily, often interpreting ambiguous or neutral situations as potentially threatening.

In the case of GAD, the individual eventually develops fundamental beliefs that the world is dangerous and that he or she is unable to handle adversity. Worry becomes the primary strategy to cope with perceived threats as the individual attempts to gain control over potential threats as well as spiraling tension and anxious arousal. Failed attempts to gain control lead to distorted cognitive processing, which inhibits effective problem-solving and constructive action. Incorporating aspects of the worry theory described below (Borkovec, Alcaine, & Behar 2004), the avoidance of worry-related images is believed to restrict autonomic response, and the worry process is negatively reinforced by the absence of catastrophic outcomes. Full GAD develops when this worry process becomes so chronic that associated somatic symptoms and clinically severe distress and impairment result.

## Avoidance Theory of Worry and GAD

Borkovec and colleagues (2004) proposed that worry serves a cognitive avoidance function, thereby preventing useful exposure to corrective internal and environmental information. Based on the early behavioral theory of Mowrer (1947), fears are acquired through classical conditioning and subsequently maintained via operant conditioning. Once the fear association has been established, behavioral avoidance of fear-relevant stimuli or situations is negatively reinforced by the reduction of immediate distress. However, overt behavioral forms of avoidance are not always necessary to maintain anxious meanings. Cognitive escape or avoidance, such as imagining oneself avoiding the feared situation, may serve the same purpose as overt behavioral avoidance even when actual behavioral avoidance is not possible (Borkovec 1979). Borkovec and colleagues suggested that worry represents another form of cognitive avoidance, which prevents the emotional processing of feared material much like behavioral avoidance of snakes prevents the effective processing of fear among individuals with snake phobia. Based on years of programmatic research, Borkovec and colleagues proposed that worry serves to avoid several unwanted experiences: aversive images, physiological arousal, future bad events or outcomes, and possibly, intense painful emotion related to past trauma and/or social and interpersonal factors. Indeed, worry is comprised largely of verbal-linguistic thought and very little visual imagery (e.g., Borkovec & Inz 1990). Imagination of emotional material evokes substantially greater physiological and emotional responses than verbal-linguistic thinking about such material (Vrana, Cuthbert, & Lang 1986). Furthermore, worry suppresses physiological responding to fearful imagery while maintaining subjective anxiety (Borkovec & Hu 1990; Borkovec, Lyonfields, Wiser, & Diehl 1993). For these reasons, Craske and Hazlett-Stevens (2002) suggested that worry may serve a cognitive avoidance function in other anxiety disorders besides GAD. We further posited that the diffuse and pervasive worry characterizing GAD develops from fundamental beliefs of personal incompetence and generalized fears of failure.

In addition to avoidance of aversive internal experiences, Borkovec and colleagues (2004) suggested that worry also may serve to avoid actual environmental events. Human beings possess a unique capacity to think ahead and anticipate future events, allowing them to identify ways of influencing the likelihood of both wanted and unwanted events. In other words, contemplating the future often leads to preemptive problem-solving behavior and prevention of threat. When this cognitive strategy is misapplied routinely, such as when no real threat exists or when the problem at hand is vaguely defined, this worry process still might be negatively reinforced by the absence of disaster. If individuals falsely attribute the absence of bad outcomes to their previous engagement in worry, they will continue to rely on worry as a perceived means to avoid additional threats in the future. The more the individual worries, the less opportunity he or she has to experience what would have happened in the absence of worry. Individuals with GAD typically endorse a variety of positive beliefs about worry, considering worry an effective way to prevent bad outcomes and/or prepare for unwanted events. These positive worry beliefs are discussed in greater detail in Chap. 6.

Finally, excessive worry may have developed as a way to avoid more difficult emotional material. Although thinking about possible future threats creates subjective anxiety and distress, it also may distract individuals from more intense painful emotional experience. Individuals suffering from GAD endorsed this reason for worry more so than a nonanxious group did (Borkovec & Roemer 1995). Individuals with GAD also are more likely than their nonanxious counterparts to report past experiences such as traumatic events (Roemer, Molina, Litz, & Borkovec 1997) and insecure attachment to caregivers during childhood (Cassidy 1995; Schut, Pincus, Castonguay, Bedics, et al. 1997). Thus, many individuals with GAD may have suffered emotionally difficult events before the natural development of skills to process and cope with such events. Worry therefore emerged as a way to manage unresolved negative emotion regarding past childhood events as well as current interpersonal events.

Mennin and colleagues recently expanded upon Borkovec and colleagues' (2004) avoidance theory of worry. Their preliminary research found evidence of heightened emotional intensity, fear of emotional experience, and poor ability to manage negative emotions among individuals with GAD (Mennin, Heimberg, Turk, & Fresco 2005). According to their emotion dysregulation model (Mennin, Heimberg, Turk, & Fresco 2002; Mennin, Turk, Heimberg, & Carmin 2004), excessive worry develops as a maladaptive emotion regulation strategy to control physiological arousal and other facets of emotional experience. However, this new theory does not specify whether individuals with GAD rely on worry to regulate primary "adaptive" emotional experience, secondary "reactive" emotions, or both. Greenberg and Safran (1987) made an important distinction between authentic primary emotions, considered adaptive emotional responses to specific situations or events, and secondary reactive emotions expressed in response to more primary emotional states. According to Greenberg and Safran, cognitive-behavioral therapists typically focus on modification of secondary emotions while experiential therapists bypass secondary emotion in the service of eliciting underlying primary emotion. Future work explicating the roles of both types of emotional states in GAD could enhance our understanding and treatment of this complex anxiety condition. Do individuals with GAD worry excessively to cope with a heavy burden of unprocessed primary negative emotion? A developmental history involving an unresponsive or abusive caregiver, a cold, rejecting, or disapproving parent, or a significant personal loss might point to the origins of such primary emotion. If so, does this unprocessed underlying primary emotion lead to an excess of secondary reactive emotions, such as anxiety and anger? Perhaps individuals with GAD struggle with internal emotional experience on two counts. First, the continued presence of unprocessed primary emotion sustains high levels of secondary reactive emotions for the individual to manage on a regular basis. In addition, the very environmental conditions responsible for the initial primary emotion may have impeded normal social-emotional development, thereby preventing the individual from acquiring effective emotion regulation skills in the first place. Both processes could leave the individual with GAD at a significant disadvantage to regulate their emotional experience. Such an individual may be unable to process adaptive primary emotional responses to past and current life events, while also experiencing more intense negative secondary emotion in response to everyday stressors. Additional research is needed to examine these theoretical propositions further. If supported, future treatment for GAD might combine cognitive-behavioral procedures that help clients manage excessive worry and anxiety with experiential therapy techniques that target unprocessed primary emotion directly. Indeed, clinical researchers at Penn State (Newman, Castonguay, Borkovec, & Molnar 2004) already have headed in this direction, integrating cognitive-behavioral therapy (CBT) with experiential therapy techniques that facilitate processing of primary emotion associated with past and current interpersonal relationships.

## Chapter Summary

GAD is a complex and chronic anxiety disorder characterized by excessive and uncontrollable worry, associated somatic symptoms such as muscle tension and sleep disturbance, and clinically significant distress or functional impairment.

Diagnostic definitions of GAD were revised considerably over the course of DSM history, with the current DSM-IV recognizing GAD as an independent diagnostic entity. A lifetime prevalence estimate of 5.7% was obtained from a recent epidemiological survey conducted in the U.S. (Kessler, Berglund, et al. 2005). Comparable prevalence rates have been reported in most, but not all, epidemiological investigations conducted in other countries. GAD affects women twice as often as men, although this gender distribution was not found in a South African sample (Bhagwanjee et al. 1998). While GAD often first appears in childhood, adolescence, or early adulthood, GAD affects older adults as well. Individuals diagnosed with GAD typically receive comorbid anxiety and/or depressive disorder diagnoses, and many suffer from concurrent medical conditions.

A wide array of neurobiological, cognitive, and behavioral factors have been implicated in the etiology and maintenance of GAD. The integrative theoretical model developed by Barlow and colleagues (Barlow 1988; Roemer et al. 2002) identifies general biological and psychological vulnerabilities that may predispose and individual to an emotional disorder. Processes specific to the development of GAD include fundamental beliefs that the world is dangerous and that one is unable to cope with adversity. Worry therefore becomes the primary strategy to cope with perceived threats as the individual attempts to gain control over potential threats as well as spiraling tension and anxious arousal. The avoidance theory of worry (Borkovec et al. 2004) outlined specific ways in which individuals with GAD rely on worry as a cognitive avoidance strategy. Feared internal experiences, such as aversive imagery, physiological arousal, and intense emotion, are avoided in addition to undesirable future outcomes. Building upon this theory, Mennin and colleagues (2004) proposed that individuals with GAD suffer from deficits in emotion regulation skills and therefore engage in such cognitive avoidance maneuvers to regulate their emotional experience. Future directions exploring how individuals with GAD experience primary adaptive emotions as well as secondary reactive emotions may inform current theoretical models and further treatment development.

# Chapter 2
# GAD Treatment Research*

Of all the anxiety disorders, GAD is considered the most difficult to treat effectively (Brown, Barlow, & Liebowitz 1994). Early psychosocial interventions for anxiety disorders utilized exposure techniques, such as systematic desensitization for the treatment of phobic behavior. However, the phenomenology of GAD proved too diffuse for the application of early exposure-based treatments (Borkovec & Whisman 1996). Therefore, early GAD treatment research included anxiety management strategies targeting somatic anxiety symptoms. Relaxation training provided clients with new and effective coping responses for use whenever anxiety cues were detected. Indeed, relaxation training remains one of the standard components in cognitive-behavioral treatment for GAD today. Later GAD treatments incorporated cognitive therapy strategies targeting inflated perceptions of threat as well as imaginal exposure to internal and external anxiety cues for the purpose of coping rehearsal. Such cognitive-behavioral treatment packages have been evaluated in numerous controlled psychotherapy outcome research trials. Although GAD remains the most difficult to treat anxiety disorder, cognitive-behavioral therapy (CBT) consistently produces significant therapeutic change that persists over time. Furthermore, CBT appears superior to no treatment and to nondirective counseling.

This chapter provides a concise review of the extant GAD psychotherapy outcome research conducted over the past 23 years. Since the earliest empirical investigations of this nature in the mid 1980's, comprehensive psychosocial treatment packages addressing the various cognitive, behavioral, and psychological features of GAD have been developed and tested. Current state-of-the-art CBT for GAD continues to receive empirical support. However, these treatments do not produce clinically meaningful change for as many clients as seen in the cognitive-behavioral treatment of other anxiety disorders. Four comprehensive literature reviews and meta-analytic studies will be described (Borkovec & Whisman 1996; Gould, Otto, Pollack, & Yap 1997; Borkovec & Ruscio 2001; Gould, Safren, Washington, & Otto 2004). More recent investigations of GAD treatment effects not captured in these reviews will be presented as well. Finally, therapy outcome research examining the treatment of GAD among older adults will be discussed.

---

* This chapter was written by Larry D. Pruitt and Holly Hazlett-Stevens.

H. Hazlett-Stevens, *Psychological Approaches to Generalized Anxiety Disorder*, doi: 10.1007/978-0-387-76870-0, © Springer Science + Business Media, LLC 2008

# Initial GAD Psychotherapy Outcome Research

Several controlled therapy trials examining the efficacy of psychosocial treatments for GAD were conducted during the mid 1980's and early 1990's. In 1996, Borkovec and Whisman conducted a comprehensive review of these and other early investigations of GAD psychotherapy effects. They reported that weak experimental methodology at that time left the results of many investigations difficult to interpret. As a result, Borkovec and Whisman applied strict methodological criteria to each investigation and only included those believed to yield interpretable results. Many methodological factors were considered, including: the method of diagnosis, the use of blind assessors, whether medication use was controlled, counterbalancing of therapists, use of written protocol manuals, assessment of treatment adherence, measurement of treatment expectancy and credibility, attrition rates, and the length of follow-up periods. Eleven controlled outcome investigations meeting the minimal methodological standards set by the authors were included. Twelve other studies were excluded, largely because of limitations in diagnostic assessment procedures and/or ambiguities in diagnostic inclusion criteria.

## *Study Characteristics*

Of the eleven investigations reviewed by Borkovec and Whisman (1996), GAD diagnosis was established with Diagnostic and Statistical Manual (DSM) criteria in seven of the eleven projects, Research Diagnostic Criteria (RDC) were applied in two studies, and an additional two studies used both methods. Blind assessors were involved in seven of the studies, but were not included in two. Blind assessment was considered not applicable in an additional two studies. For investigations in which medication use was applicable, patient medication usage was balanced in two investigations, left unchecked in one study, and unknown in four studies. To minimize any effects specific to the therapist, rather than the treatment, the authors examined whether each investigation counterbalanced therapists across therapy conditions. Only two studies employed this approach. Five investigations did not counterbalance therapists, and this methodological design feature either was not applicable or was not mentioned in four studies. Treatment adherence and client expectancies of treatment were both assessed in seven of the eleven studies. Of the entire list of eleven investigations, attrition rates ranged from 0% to 37.5% with a mean of 11.2%. Final follow-up assessments were conducted an average of 11.2 months after the end of treatment.

## *Sample Characteristics and Treatment Features*

The mean age of the clients who participated in these eleven studies was 36 years, consisting of 383 women (65.1%) and 205 men (34.9%). The average duration of GAD symptoms was 5.5 years. Four studies included clients who were concurrently maintained on a fixed dosage of medication. Among these four studies, 40.4% of clients were taking psychoactive medication. With regard to treatment, the average number of sessions was 10.3 with a range from 4 to 18. Treatment sessions were on average 64.1 min in length but ranged from 40 to 120 min. An average of 5.5 therapists provided treatment, but the number of therapists ranged from 2 to 16. The types of therapists varied and included professional clinicians, a mix of clinicians and graduate students, graduate students only, and, in the case of one investigation, psychiatric nurses.

## Treatment Outcome Results

Borkovec and Whisman (1996) first examined within-group results reported in the eleven reviewed investigations. Each active psychosocial treatment produced significant improvement pre to post treatment on all outcome measures. These active psychosocial treatments included cognitive-behavior therapy, anxiety management training, cognitive therapy alone, behavior therapy alone, and applied relaxation. Nonspecific control conditions, including nondirective counseling, psychosocial placebo, pill placebo, and diazepam, yielded significant changes on fewer measures than the active treatments. No-treatment control conditions (six studies) did not result in changes over time, suggesting that spontaneous remission did not account for the effects observed in the other conditions. Furthermore, two investigations (Butler, Fennell, Robson, & Gelder 1991; Barlow, Rapee, & Brown 1992) reported decreased psychoactive medication use among active treatment condition participants. Therapy gains associated with behavioral and cognitive-behavioral interventions maintained at follow-up on most measures, and in two studies, further improvement on some measures was reported. Improvements resulting from nonspecific therapy conditions were shorter-lived, with most of these clients experiencing some degree of relapse by the follow-up assessment. Treatment gains resulting from placebo conditions also tended not to persist. Borkovec and Whisman concluded that improvement of GAD is unlikely to occur without treatment and that improvements associated with the active psychosocial interventions could not be attributed only to nonspecific factors.

Active psychosocial interventions were compared to control conditions directly with between-group statistical comparisons. In all of the six investigations including a no-treatment condition, the active psychosocial treatment resulted in greater improvement than the no-treatment condition on all or most measures. Results from studies comparing cognitive-behavioral or behavioral therapies to nonspecific control conditions were less clear. Generally these comparisons revealed that active cognitive-behavioral or behavioral interventions were superior to nonspecific control conditions on some measures. While these results certainly were promising, Borkovec and Whisman (1996) cautioned that strong between-group effects were not found often. Across all treatment conditions, CBT did produce the largest degree of change on measures of anxiety and depression when calculated within-group effect sizes were compared in a meta-analysis. Effect sizes associated with CBT interventions also were significantly larger than those associated with all other psychosocial interventions. When CBT was examined in terms of clinically significant change (a return to within one standard deviation of the mean of the normal population), 75% of the studies reported long-term maintenance or gains toward achieving clinically significant change. However, four of six investigations comparing active treatment conditions to each other (Barlow et al. 1992; White, Keenan, & Brooks 1992; Borkovec & Costello 1993; Borkovec & Mathews 1988) found no between-group differences when comparing: 1) cognitive therapy to applied relaxation, 2) cognitive therapy alone to behavior therapy alone to CBT, 3) applied relaxation to applied relaxation plus cognitive therapy and self-control desensitization, and 4) cognitive therapy plus relaxation to self-control desensitization plus relaxation to non-directive therapy plus relaxation. Two of the six studies did find some significant group differences. Butler et al. (1991) found that CBT was superior to behavior therapy alone on some measures, and Borkovec, Mathews, Chambers, Ebrahimi, et al. (1987) found that cognitive therapy plus relaxation was superior to non-directive therapy plus relaxation on some measures. Borkovec and Whisman concluded that these last two studies may suggest a potential incremental effect for cognitive therapy when combined with other behavioral interventions such as relaxation training.

## *Summary of Preliminary Research Findings*

According to the review conducted by Borkovec and Whisman (1996), CBT interventions yielded larger within-group effect sizes and greater clinically significant change, both at the end of treatment and over a one-year follow-up period, than other psychosocial treatments for GAD. CBT was also associated with lower dropout rates and larger reductions in psychoactive medication use during and after treatment. Borkovec and Whisman concluded that the combination of cognitive therapy, behavior therapy and relaxation techniques, and self-control desensitization, consisting of imaginal exposure and coping rehearsal procedures, is most likely to produce long-term improvement in both the somatic and cognitive features of GAD. Indeed, updated procedures for each of these recommended therapy components are provided in this book. However, a variety of empirical questions remain. Which of these treatment components are most important? In combination they appear to work, but are all components needed to achieve desired therapeutic change? Are all therapy components equally essential, or are some components more effective than others? Clarifying the role of nonspecific factors and isolating the specific effects of individual treatment components both would enhance our understanding of why cognitive-behavioral GAD treatment works.

# Cognitive-Behavioral and Pharmacological Treatment Research

The review and meta-analysis conducted by Borkovec and Whisman (1996) included investigations of psychosocial treatment effects only. Around that same time, Gould et al. (1997) conducted a meta-analytic review of controlled trials including both CBT and pharmacotherapy treatment for GAD. This review was much broader in scope, examining 35 investigations. A total of 61 individual treatment comparisons were available from research conducted between 1974 and 1996. Thus, this was the first meta-analysis comparing CBT to pharmacological interventions for GAD. Gould et al. included both published and unpublished "in press" research projects in their meta-analytic investigation.

## *Inclusion Criteria and Methodological Considerations*

Gould et al. (1997) limited their analysis to investigations with a control group so they could compute a precise between-group effect size for each intervention. Acceptable control conditions included no treatment, wait list, or pill/psychological placebo. Participants either met DSM diagnostic criteria for GAD or would have met those criteria had they been applied to the sample. Randomization of participants to condition was not set as a specific inclusion criterion, but this methodological characteristic was typical among the investigations included. Concurrent medication use was not an exclusion criterion, but rather was considered a variable of interest.

## *CBT Outcome Results*

Each treatment condition was classified as either cognitive-behavioral or pharmacological. Cognitive-behavioral treatments included cognitive restructuring, situational exposure, imaginal exposure, interoceptive exposure, systematic desensitization, relaxation training, relaxation with biofeedback, anxiety management training, or any combination thereof. The mean effect size (ES) across all CBT interventions was 0.70 for anxiety measures and 0.77 for symptoms of depression, both of which were statistically significant when compared to no treatment. According to Cohen (1988), an ES of 0.2 is considered a small effect, an ES of 0.5 reflects a medium-sized effect, and an ES of 0.8 is a large effect. The effect size calculated when cognitive therapy interventions were examined alone, based on three studies, was 0.59. For behavior therapy alone, also based on three studies, the calculated effect size was 0.51. Cognitive and behavioral strategies were combined in eight investigations, resulting in a CBT treatment package effect size of 0.91. When used as independent treatment strategies, anxiety management training and relaxation training had effect sizes of 0.91 and 0.64 respectively. Relaxation with biofeedback had the lowest effect size of 0.34 and was significantly lower than combined CBT strategies. The mean attrition rate for CBT studies was 10.6%. With regard to treatment format, there were no statistical differences between the effect sizes of group interventions (0.66) versus individual interventions (0.81). No differences were found with regard to length of treatment, as CBT treatments ranged from 4 to 15 hours of intervention with a mean of 9.5 clinical hours.

## Pharmacotherapy Outcome Results

Pharmacological interventions included all drugs that had been approved by the United States Food and Drug Administration for the treatment of GAD as well as agents that had not received such approval but were commonly prescribed for GAD. The 24 trials selected for meta-analysis included thirty-nine separate interventions, and all twenty-four investigations utilized pill placebo control conditions. The active pharmacotherapy interventions yielded an overall effect size of 0.60 for symptoms of anxiety and an overall effect size of 0.46 for depressive symptoms. The associated attrition rate was 15.2%. Interventions employing benzodiazepines were the most common, included in 23 of the studies. When examined in isolation, these medications produced an overall effect size of 0.70 and a 13.1% drop-out rate. Investigations using diazepam specifically were the second most common type of pharmacologic investigation, represented by eleven studies. This intervention produced the largest effect size (0.76) but also the highest dropout rate (16.9%) of the benzodiazepine class. Trials examining Lorazepam, Alprazolam, Bromazepam, and buspirone yielded effect sizes of 0.66, 0.44, 0.61, 0.39 respectively, with dropout rates ranging from 8% to 16.8%. Antidepressant medications were examined in three studies, resulting in an effect size of 0.57 and one-third of participants (33.5%) dropping out of treatment.

## Comparisons Between CBT and Pharmacological Treatments

When the overarching intervention categories of CBT (ES = 0.70) and pharmacotherapy (ES = 0.60) were compared, no significant differences in anxiety symptom reduction were found between the two treatment modalities. In addition, no differences in attrition rates were found (10.6% for CBT, 15.2% for pharmacotherapy). However, Gould et al. (1997) found that CBT interventions (ES = 0.77) were superior to pharmacological interventions (ES = 0.46) in the reduction of depressive symptomatology, although only three of the pharmacology trials measured depression. Gould and colleagues warned that the effect sizes associated with CBT inadvertently may have been inflated by the use of control groups that were less stringent than the pill placebo control groups found in pharmacology trials.

Nevertheless, CBT interventions were associated with maintenance of treatment gains at least 6 months later. Long-term effects of the pharmacological interventions often were not examined, although some evidence of lost treatment gains following discontinuation of diazepam was found. Additional concerns might be raised for medication treatment of women during their childbearing years, as the effects of these agents on the fetus are unknown. Interestingly, over 60% of the patients included in this meta-analytic review were women.

## Recent GAD Treatment Outcome Meta-Analysis Results

Both research groups described above recently updated their reviews, including newer investigations published since the mid 1990's. Borkovec and Ruscio (2001) re-analyzed controlled GAD psychotherapy outcome investigation results, comparing CBT treatment packages to individual cognitive and behavioral components as well as to no-treatment and nonspecific control conditions. In 2004, Gould and colleagues conducted a new meta-analysis containing only those investigations which included some form of cognitive-behavioral treatment. Both of these recent meta-analytic investigations provided a more sophisticated and complete picture of CBT effects in the treatment of GAD.

### *Updated Psychotherapy Outcome Meta-Analytic Review Results*

Borkovec and Ruscio (2001) conducted a meta-analytic review of 13 controlled clinical trials of CBT for GAD. They selected the same eleven investigations included in the earlier Borkovec and Whisman (1996) review and added two clinical trials conducted since the original review. Many rigorous methodological characteristics of these 13 investigations were identified. Eight of the thirteen studies included diagnostic reliability checks, and three of these eight further included independent diagnostic interviews for every client to exclude false positive cases. Further methodological considerations such as blind assessors, balancing therapist caseload to prevent therapist effects (8 studies), strict treatment protocols (9 studies), and protocol adherence checks (8 studies) were also reported. Additionally, nine of the thirteen studies assessed nonspecific factors, including client perceptions of treatment credibility and outcome expectancies. Six of the studies reviewed allowed clients with concurrent medication use to participate, but most required clients to maintain their current dosage throughout the treatment period. Participants were, on average, in their late thirties, and approximately two-thirds were women. The average duration of GAD symptoms was 7 years. Treatment involved an average of 10.6 therapy sessions, and session length averaged 69 min.

Borkovec and Ruscio (2001) classified each of the treatment conditions into four groups: CBT package interventions, cognitive therapy only or behavior therapy only, pill placebo or non-cognitive/behavioral alternative treatment (e.g., psychodynamic therapy, nondirective counseling/supportive listening, pharmacotherapy), and waiting-list or no treatment. As expected, CBT conditions produced the largest within-group effect sizes on both anxiety and depression measures. The next largest effect sizes were found for the alternative treatments, followed by the single-component cognitive or behavioral treatments. Not surprisingly, waiting-list and no treatment conditions did not produce changes over time. Unlike the previous Borkovec and Whisman (1996) review, Borkovec and Ruscio also calculated between-group effect sizes so that the effects of CBT could be contrasted with control condition effects. This meta-analysis revealed that CBT package treatments were superior to no treatment in all investigations (mean ES = 1.09 on anxiety measures post-treatment, mean ES = 0.92 on depression measures post-treatment). CBT also appeared superior to nonspecific or alternative treatment conditions post-treatment in 82% of the studies that examined this comparison (mean ES = 0.71 for anxiety, mean ES = 0.66 for depression). Finally, CBT outperformed cognitive therapy and behavior therapy single components in 20% of comparisons at post-treatment assessment (mean ES = 0.26 for both anxiety and depression measures separately). Fortunately, all 13 investigations reviewed included follow-up assessments, either 6 months or 12 months after treatment ended. Clinical improvements associated with active treatments were consistently maintained, or improved upon, at follow-up. Between-group effect sizes calculated with follow-up assessment data changed in opposing directions, depending on which treatments were selected for comparison. CBT appeared even more superior to cognitive or behavior therapy single component treatments at follow-up (mean ES = 0.54 for anxiety measures and mean ES = 0.45 for depression measures) than at post-treatment. However, effects sizes were lower at follow-up than at post-treatment when CBT was compared to placebo and alternative control treatments (mean ES = 0.30 for anxiety and mean ES = 0.21 for depression). Borkovec and Ruscio suggested that these effect size reductions may have been due to the fact that clients assigned to placebo conditions were more likely to seek additional treatment between post-treatment and follow-up assessment.

## *Updated CBT Meta-Analytic Review Results*

Most recently, Gould et al. (2004) conducted a meta-analysis using similar methods to their original 1997 meta-analytic review. However, this updated review contained only 16 investigations because Gould and colleagues selected only those studies which included some form of cognitive-behavioral treatment. Thirteen of these investigations were included in their 1997 meta-analysis, and Gould et al. identified three additional studies conducted since their original review. Similar to the results of their previous meta-analysis, Gould et al. (2004) found a mean ES for all forms of CBT of 0.73 for anxiety measures and 0.77 for depression measures. Both of these effect size statistics were statistically significant when compared against the null hypothesis predicting no increase in efficacy relative to the control conditions. When types of CBT interventions were examined further, CBT package treatments yielded a mean ES on anxiety measures of 0.90 and anxiety management training resulted in an average anxiety ES of 0.91. Relaxation training alone produced a mean ES of 0.64, cognitive therapy alone produced an average ES of 0.59, and interventions consisting of only behavior therapy techniques yielded a mean effect size of 0.51. Relaxation training combined with biofeedback produced a relatively small mean ES of 0.34. Two of the reviewed studies also included the pharmacological treatment diazepam, resulting in an average ES of 0.41 when compared to a pill placebo. CBT in these two studies produced a mean effect size of 1.26 when compared to pill placebo. Furthermore, the combination of CBT and diazepam greatly enhanced the effects of diazepam alone, but only appeared to increase the effects of CBT alone slightly.

Gould and colleagues concluded that CBT package treatments seem to produce the strongest treatment effects and may offer some advantage over single component cognitive or behavioral treatments. However, the clinical significance associated with such statistically significant findings is more difficult to ascertain. One of the earlier investigations reviewed (Butler et al. 1991) found that only 32% of clients who received CBT and 16% of clients who received behavior therapy met criteria for high end-state functioning. On the other hand, the more recent Ladouceur, Dugas, Freeston, Léger, et al. (2000) investigation found that 77% of participants no longer met GAD diagnostic criteria after CBT treatment ended. Furthermore, 62% of clients met additional high end-state functioning criteria. Most treatment gains were maintained at 6-month and at 12-month follow-up. The CBT intervention developed by Ladouceur and colleagues targeted core cognitive features including intolerance of uncertainty, worry beliefs, poor problem-solving orientation, and cognitive avoidance, and this particular CBT protocol also appears effective when delivered in a group format (Dugas, Ladouceur, Léger, Freeston, et al. 2003). In short, while various CBT treatments are likely to lead to clinical improvement, clients receiving these treatments do not always experience full recovery.

## Additional GAD Treatment Research

A few recent GAD psychotherapy outcome investigations were not captured in the meta-analytic reviews described above. In their most recent randomized controlled trial of CBT, Borkovec and colleagues compared their full CBT package treatment to its two individual components (Borkovec, Newman, Pincus, & Lytle 2002). Öst and Breitholtz (2000) compared applied relaxation to cognitive therapy using a randomized design, but found little evidence that one treatment component was superior to the other. Arntz (2003) conducted a similar investigation and found similar results. However, methodological limitations leave some of the results obtained from these component control investigations difficult to interpret. Newer forms of treatment attempt to improve outcomes for individuals suffering from GAD further, and preliminary research on these new treatment developments are promising.

## Component Analysis of CBT for GAD

In their most recent investigation, Borkovec and colleagues (2002) randomly assigned treatment-seeking participants diagnosed with GAD to one of three therapy conditions: cognitive therapy alone, applied relaxation with self-control desensitization, and a CBT package treatment including all of these components. A total of 76 clients received 14 weeks of individual therapy and were followed for a two-year follow-up period. All three therapy conditions produced strong therapeutic effects, but no group differences were found immediately following treatment or at any of the follow-up assessment periods. In addition, approximately half of these clients met stringent criteria for high end-state functioning at the end of treatment, many of whom maintained these gains over the two-year follow-up period. For example, over 56% of clients who received the full CBT package treatment met high end-state functioning criteria following treatment and 6 months later. This figure dropped to 43% 1 year after treatment and to 38% 2 years after treatment. Results from a measure of interpersonal problems suggested that interpersonal behavior may be an important additional treatment target for individuals with GAD. Neither CBT nor its individual components appeared to improve interpersonal functioning.

Borkovec and colleagues concluded that while CBT provides clinically significant benefit to many clients, further treatment development beyond the intrapersonally-oriented CBT approach is needed. Borkovec, Newman, and Castonguay (2003) have since integrated interpersonal and experiential therapy components into their current CBT for GAD. Preliminary research results for their newly developed "interpersonal/ emotional processing" (I/EP) treatment for GAD are encouraging (Newman, Castonguay, Borkovec, & Molnar 2004). In an open trial, 18 clients meeting GAD criteria were treated with 15 sessions of this integrative treatment. Results suggested that interpersonal treatment components can be added to CBT successfully while maintaining therapeutic alliance and therapist credibility. Within-group effect sizes for treatment outcome were slightly larger than those found for traditional CBT. Currently, a large clinical trial is underway to examine the efficacy of this treatment further.

## Comparisons Between Applied Relaxation and Cognitive Therapy

Öst and Breitholtz (2000) randomly assigned 36 treatment-seeking clients diagnosed with GAD to either applied relaxation or cognitive therapy treatment conditions. Clients received twelve sessions of individual therapy and were re-assessed following treatment and at one-year follow-up. Both treatments resulted in large clinical improvements that were maintained, and sometimes even furthered, 1 year later. No group differences on any of the outcome measures were found, perhaps because of the small sample size. Sixty-two percent of the cognitive therapy group met clinically significant change criteria post-treatment. By the 1-year follow-up period, this figure dropped to 56%. Among applied relaxation group participants, 53% met clinical significance criteria following treatment, and this figure increased to 67% at the follow-up assessment.

In a second study of this nature, Arntz (2003) randomly assigned 45 clients diagnosed with GAD to twelve sessions of either applied relaxation or cognitive therapy treatment. As expected, both treatments yielded improvements on clinical variables including measures of trait anxiety, fear, and depression. Between-group analyses demonstrated greater improvement for the applied relaxation group following treatment, but the two groups were equivalent at 6-month follow-up. At that time, 53% of clients who received applied relaxation and 55% of clients who received cognitive therapy had obtained clinically significant recovery.

## *Summary of Recent Research Findings and Future Directions*

Results from these three investigations further support the efficacy of CBT, both as a package treatment and when broken down into its separate components. These results did not provide additional support for the combination of multiple cognitive and behavioral treatment components. However, important methodological factors should be considered when interpreting these results. Psychotherapy outcome research trials tend to involve relatively small sample sizes. This limitation may not allow for sufficient statistical power to detect small incremental effects of each therapy component. Indeed, Borkovec et al. (2002) argued that the lack of group differences found in their investigation may be attributed to the strength of the therapeutic effects generated by each therapy component condition. The more powerful meta-analytic statistical procedures utilized by Borkovec and Ruscio (2001) and by Gould et al. (2004) addressed this limitation. Results from both of those investigations did provide empirical support for the combination of therapy components seen in CBT package treatments. Despite significant advances in GAD treatment development, a large minority of clients do not reach high levels of end-state functioning. Further treatment development targeting additional clinical features, such as problematic interpersonal behavior patterns, may increase the efficacy of GAD treatment even more.

Newer psychosocial treatments for GAD have departed from traditional CBT procedures, and preliminary research support for these treatments has become available. For example, a Supportive-Expressive psychodynamic therapy developed specifically for GAD targets cognition and behavior surrounding interpersonal themes such as obtaining love, security, stability, or protection from others (Crits-Christoph, Crits-Christoph, Wolf-Palacio, Fichter, & Rudick 1995). This psychotherapy research group tested the effects of their treatment in an open trial investigation (Crits-Christoph, Connolly, Azarian, Crits-Christoph, & Shappell 1996). A total of 26 treatment-seeking clients diagnosed with GAD were included. Therapists were trained according to a treatment manual, and therapists successfully adhered to this therapy protocol with competence and fidelity. Clients demonstrated significant improvement on measures of anxiety, worry, depression, and interpersonal problems.

A meta-cognitive treatment for GAD recently received empirical support from an open trial as well. Wells and King (2005) provided this newly developed therapy to ten clients meeting DSM-IV diagnostic criteria for GAD. Clients attended a range of three to twelve sessions targeting meta-cognitive factors such as counter-productive thought control strategies and negative beliefs about worry itself. Significant improvements following treatment were reported for all clients, and these improvements were maintained at 6- and 12- month follow-up for nine of the ten clients. In a final open trial conducted by Roemer and Orsillo (2007), sixteen clients diagnosed with GAD completed sixteen sessions of individual acceptance-based behavior therapy. This treatment integrated mindfulness training (Segal, Williams, & Teasdale 2002), Acceptance and Commitment Therapy (ACT; Hayes, Strosahl, & Wilson 1999) and Dialectical Behavior Therapy (DBT; Linehan 1993) into an existing CBT treatment protocol based on the work of Borkovec and colleagues (2002). Significant improvements were found on a clinician-rated GAD symptom severity measure as well as self-report measures of anxiety, depression, experiential avoidance, and quality of life. Successful case study results were reported following Emotion Regulation Therapy (ERT; Mennin 2004), an integra-tive treatment that teaches clients adaptive emotion regulation skills and guides clients toward confrontation of core issues with experiential therapy techniques. Thus, a number of new treatments for GAD expand upon the traditional cognitive-behavioral approach. Additional information about the efficacy of these new interventions will become available as further treatment outcome research is conducted.

## GAD Treatment for Older Adults

Unfortunately, much of GAD outcome research just described cannot be generalized readily to individuals outside the ages of 18–65. Not only were the majority of outcome measures originally developed for people ages 18–65, but anxiety can, and often does, present differently in child, adolescent, adult, and elderly populations (Alwahhabi 2003). Generalized anxiety disorder is one of the most frequent diagnoses among indi-viduals over age 65, and GAD is three times more common than major depression in this age group (Blazer 1997; Beekman, Bremmer, Deeg, van Balkom, et al. 1998). Nearly half of elderly persons meeting diagnostic criteria for GAD developed the dis-order later in life, but for those with an earlier symptom onset, a more severe course is typical (Le Roux, Gatz, & Wetherell 2005). Notable advances have been made in the areas of GAD treatment development and outcome research for elderly adults, although less empirical research targeting this special population is currently available.

### Early Psychotherapy Outcome Research

Early controlled clinical trials examined the efficacy of CBT for anxiety symptoms among the elderly in the absence of diagnostic assessment. In their review of this literature, Stanley and Novy (2000) found consistent empirical support for the use of CBT treatments, particularly relaxation training, among older community volunteer participants with various anxiety-related complaints. For example, Scogin, Rickard, Keith, Wilson, and McElreath (1992) compared four sessions of progressive relaxation training to an imaginal relaxation procedure. A wait-list control group was included as well. The sample consisted of 71 participants in their late sixties endorsing elevated subjective anxiety. Both relaxation conditions produced significant reductions in state anxiety levels compared to the wait-list control condition, and these gains were maintained at least 1 year following treatment (Rickard, Scogin, & Keith 1994). The attrition rate, however, was 24%, as only 54 of the original 71 participants completed treatment.

## GAD Psychotherapy Outcome Research

A few controlled therapy trials since have been conducted with older participants diagnosed with GAD. In the first investigation of this nature (Stanley, Beck, & Glassco 1996), adults aged 55–81 received either CBT or a nondirective supportive therapy control treatment. Each treatment consisted of 14 weekly small group therapy sessions. Both therapy conditions produced significant changes on self-report as well as clinician-administered measures, and therapy gains were largely maintained or improved at 6-month follow-up. However, group differences on outcome measures were not found.

In a replication and extension of their initial outcome trial, Stanley and colleagues randomized 80 older adults (age 60 or over) to group-administered CBT or a minimal contact control condition (Stanley, Beck, Novy, Averill, et al. 2003). Results from both treatment completer and intent-to-treat analyses demonstrated that clients who received CBT experienced greater improvement across a variety of outcome measures compared to the control group. Although therapy gains were maintained at one-year follow-up and 45% of clients who received CBT were classified as treatment responders, clients did not return to normative levels of functioning.

In a third randomized psychotherapy outcome investigation of CBT for late-life GAD (Wetherell, Gatz, & Craske 2003), group-administered CBT was compared to a structured discussion control therapy as well as to a wait-list control group. Both therapies proved superior to the wait-list control condition, but no differences between the two therapy conditions were found by 6-month follow-up. However, only CBT produced large effect sizes following treatment (average ES = 0.79), whereas the discussion control group therapy yielded only small to medium-sized effects (ES = 0.36).

In each of these three investigations, the CBT protocol used was based on a cognitive-behavioral treatment for GAD developed for younger adults (e.g., Craske, Barlow, & O'Leary 1992) with only slight modifications for older adults. However, treatment was conducted in a small group format. Group treatment may be ideal for this population given that older adults frequently experience losses in their social networks (Wetherell, Hopko, Diefenbach, Averill, et al. 2005). Although group CBT treatments generally appear effective for older adults suffering from GAD, the impact of such treatments may be significantly reduced among clients facing con-current medical problems (Radley, Redston, Bates, Pontefract, & Lindesay 1997). Individual CBT also may be effective for older adults diagnosed with GAD. In a single-case experimental multiple-baseline design, Ladouceur and colleagues treated eight adults (age 60–71) diagnosed with GAD using an adapted version of their CBT protocol (Ladouceur, Léger, Dugas, & Freeston 2004). Seven of the eight participants improved significantly by the end of treatment, and these gains were maintained at six and 12-month follow-up.

## *Other Treatment-Related Research*

Researchers also have identified specific variables that may be related to positive treatment response among older adults (Wetherell et al. 2005). Data from the three psychotherapy outcome projects described above were pooled and analyzed for inves-tigation of outcome predictors (Stanley et al. 1996, 2003; Wetherell et al. 2003), result-ing in a total sample of 65 adults with a mean age of 67 years. All three of these projects utilized the same treatment manual and inclusion/exclusion criteria. Demographic, clinical, treatment, and outcome variables were similar across all three projects. The CBT intervention was delivered in a group format and included psychoeducation, relaxation strategies, imaginal exposure, cognitive restructuring, and behavior modification. Results suggested that initial GAD severity, the presence of co-morbid conditions, and degree of engagement in homework exercises predicted treatment-related improvement in GAD severity, especially at 6-month follow-up.

Blazer (1997) suggested that in addition to standard CBT components, clinicians should consider including memory training when treating the elderly. Memory training is an intervention designed to improve memory or to adapt to existing memory difficulties (Yesavage, Sheikh, Tanke, & Hill 1988). Indeed, some research supports the modification of traditional CBT procedures when treating elderly cli-ents. In a series of studies, Mohlman, Gorenstein, Kleber, De Jesus, et al. (2003) examined the effects of an individual CBT treatment specifically suited to older adults. This treatment included memory and learning aids, homework reminders, and weekly review sessions. Both standard CBT and enhanced CBT treatments resulted in decreased GAD frequency and severity. However, the enhanced CBT produced reductions on a broader variety of outcome measures than the standard CBT. Furthermore, the enhanced CBT produced greater effect sizes than the stand-ard CBT when each active treatment was compared to a wait list control condition. Fifty percent of clients treated with standard CBT no longer met diagnostic criteria at the end of treatment, whereas 86% of clients who received the enhanced CBT no longer met criteria. Another modified CBT protocol was designed to accommodate sensory and cognitive challenges that are often present for older clients (Stanley, Hopko, Diefenbach, Bourland, et al. 2003). In a small pilot investigation, clients who received this modified CBT treatment showed statistically significant improvement when compared to clients in a treatment-as-usual control group.

Older adults taking anxiolytic medication for their anxiety symptoms may benefit from the combination of CBT and a medical management for medication taper intervention. Gorenstein, Kleber, Mohlman, De Jesus, et al. (2005) developed this intervention with the aim of reducing anxiety symptoms as well as anxiolytic medication dependence. Older adults who completed this combination intervention experienced greater improvements on psychological measures than clients randomized to a medical management only condition, and some of these gains were maintained at 6-month follow-up. Both client groups significantly reduced their medication usage. Gorenstein and colleagues concluded that CBT appears to alleviate anxiety symptoms, even as clients take steps to reduce anxiolytic medication.

A final possible treatment modification when working with elderly clients involves conducting treatment in the client's home. This option allows clients who are disabled or unable to travel access to treatment. Barrowclough, King, Colville, Russell et al. (2001) compared a standard CBT delivered in the home to a supportive counseling and empathetic listening control treatment. Fifty-five patients with a mean age of 72 meeting diagnostic criteria for GAD, panic disorder, social phobia, or anxiety disorder NOS were treated with 16 1-hour individual sessions. Clients in the CBT condition improved significantly more than clients randomized to the supportive counseling condition on measures of anxiety and depression immediately after treatment and at 1-year follow-up.

Taken together, these empirical research results suggest that older adults with GAD may benefit from a cognitive-behavioral treatment approach and that modifications to standard CBT protocols may increase the efficacy of these treatments further. Future efforts to improve CBT outcomes for older adults are certainly needed, however, as many older clients remain within the clinical range on psychopathology measures at the conclusion of treatment.

# Chapter Summary

Many randomized controlled clinical trials have examined the efficacy of CBT for GAD over the past couple of decades. In their 1996 review, Borkovec and Whisman concluded that cognitive-behavioral treatments consistently produce significant therapeutic gains which typically are maintained at follow-up. The results of a meta-analysis conducted by Gould and colleagues (1997) suggested that CBT and pharmacotherapy yield roughly equivalent outcomes in the short term, but only the benefits associated with CBT maintain through follow-up periods. An updated meta-analysis of GAD psychotherapy outcome research (Borkovec & Ruscio 2001) further found that CBT consistently proved superior to no treatment and to nonspecific control conditions. CBT sometimes outperformed single cognitive or behavioral component treatments. In their updated meta-analysis of CBT for GAD research, Gould and colleagues (2004) also reported that CBT package treatments seem to produce the strongest treatment effects and may offer some advantage over single component cognitive or behavioral treatments. However, the clinical significance associated with such statistically significant findings is difficult to ascertain, and many clients with GAD experience some benefit from CBT without returning to high levels of end-state functioning.

More recent treatment research (Borkovec et al. 2002) identified additional clinical problems associated with GAD that might be targeted in future psychotherapy protocols. This research group has integrated experiential and interpersonal therapy techniques into their traditional CBT for GAD with promising results (Newman et al. 2004). An interpersonally-oriented brief psychodynamic treatment (Crits-Christoph et al. 1996), a meta-cognitive therapy (Wells & King 2005), and an acceptance-based behavior therapy (Roemer & Orsillo 2007) also are gaining preliminary empirical support.

Most GAD treatment research was conducted with adult samples in the 18–65 age range. However, a growing interest in the nature and treatment of GAD among older adults has emerged. A few psychotherapy outcome investigations support the use of CBT protocols in the treatment of older adults. These outcomes might be further improved with slight modifications such as memory training, learning aids, homework reminders, weekly review sessions, and delivery of therapy sessions in the home.

Despite its limitations, CBT remains the psychosocial intervention for GAD with the greatest amount of empirical support. The combination of psychoeducation, applied relaxation training, cognitive therapy, and behavioral and imaginal exposure treatment components consistently has helped individuals suffering from this difficult to treat anxiety disorder. Nevertheless, additional treatment development efforts are needed to improve the efficacy of psychotherapy for GAD further. The forthcoming chapters of this book explain each of these cognitive-behavioral procedures in great detail, largely based upon the CBT for GAD developed by Borkovec and colleagues (2002). Additional suggestions for the integration of adjunct therapy techniques that may enhance the efficacy of traditional CBT are provided throughout these chapters as well.

# Chapter 3
# Assessment Procedures and Treatment Planning

A variety of clinical assessment methods aid clinicians with diagnosis and treatment planning. Comprehensive assessment extends beyond determining which GAD diagnostic criteria and associated symptoms are present. Clinicians also evaluate any comorbid psychological and medical conditions, interpersonal functioning and social support systems, and idiosyncratic cognitive and behavioral patterns. Assessment typically commences with a clinical interview, serving as a diagnostic assessment tool as well as a means for gathering additional information needed for treatment planning. This chapter begins with a discussion of diagnostic assessment procedures and a review of available clinician-administered diagnostic interviews. Selected self-report measures of important constructs believed to underlie GAD symptoms are presented next. Finally, this chapter concludes with a description of the treatment planning process, including specific guidelines for incorporating assessment information into a personalized treatment plan.

## Diagnostic Assessment

Clinical evaluation often begins with a formal assessment of GAD symptoms and associated features. Information regarding specific symptoms is collected to determine whether DSM-IV diagnostic criteria are met. This diagnostic information also guides clinicians in their selection of an initial treatment approach and their construction of a treatment plan. Diagnostic interviews range from an unstructured consultation to a highly structured series of verbatim interview questions. Both extremes carry notable advantages and disadvantages; the degree of structure required largely depends upon the setting in which diagnostic interviews are conducted. Regardless of the diagnostic interview style, accurate diagnosis requires careful consideration of GAD diagnostic criteria and several differential diagnostic issues.

H. Hazlett-Stevens, *Psychological Approaches to Generalized Anxiety Disorder,*
doi: 10.1007/978-0-387-76870-0, © Springer Science + Business Media, LLC 2008

## *Diagnostic Considerations*

As reviewed in Chap. 1, DSM-IV GAD diagnosis requires excessive anxiety and worry during a majority of the time over the past 6 months. The worry is experienced as difficult to control and covers a range of events or activities. At least three of six associated symptoms are present, some of which also must occur most of the time over the past 6 months. The anxiety, worry, and related symptoms cause significant functional impairment or distress. Finally, the anxiety and worry are not limited to another Axis I disorder and are not due to the direct physiological effects of substance use or a medical condition.

Clinicians are faced with the initial diagnostic decision of whether or not an individual's worry and anxiety are truly excessive. Distinguishing normal from pathological worry can be difficult, as many people endorse worrying from time to time. Questions about the frequency of each worry topic, the emotional intensity accompanying the worry, and whether the distress caused by the worry seems out of proportion to the importance of the worry topic are often helpful. If the worry is frequent, continuous, and tends to generate anxiety and subjective distress that builds over the course of the day, the excessiveness criterion has probably been met. Many people live with clinically significant GAD symptoms throughout much of their lives without ever seeking help. Given the chronic course of GAD, some individuals might not endorse questions about clinically significant distress or functional impairment at first. Clinicians often need to ask probing questions about how worry and anxiety have affected different areas of an individual's life (e.g., relationships, work performance and job selection, leisure activities) as well as the person's overall quality of life.

Once the clinician concludes that an individual is suffering from clinically severe GAD symptoms, the nature and focus of worry content must be considered. DSM-IV requires that the worry and anxiety is about a "number" of events or activities and is not confined to the features of another Axis I disorder. For a valid GAD diagnosis to be made, the worry and anxiety must be diffuse and not merely stem from an underlying circumscribed fear. Thus, clinicians must ask about the nature of an individual's worry to determine whether symptoms can be better accounted for by another diagnosis. Questions such as "What exactly are you concerned about when you worry about work?" or "What sorts of things do you fear could happen when you're worrying about your job?" can uncover explicit fears consistent with a different Axis I diagnosis. Many anxiety and related mental disorders are characterized by excessive worry: panic disordered individuals worry about unexpected panic attacks; social anxiety disordered individuals worry about embarrassment and negative evaluation; eating disordered individuals worry about weight gain; and individuals with various somatoform disorders worry about their physical health, functioning, or appearance. In contrast, the worry seen in GAD encompasses a variety of daily matters with several potential negative outcomes. Pointed differential diagnostic questions should be asked to clarify whether a client's anxiety and worry are better accounted for by another disorder.

Differential diagnosis between obsessive-compulsive disorder (OCD) and GAD is often fairly straightforward. The DSM-IV draws a relatively clear distinction between obsessions and worry. Obsessions are considered ego-dystonic cognitive intrusions in the form of urges, impulses, or images rather than ego-syntonic self-talk about everyday problems. In addition to the obsessions required for OCD diagnosis, OCD individuals often experience excessive OCD-related worry in response to their obsessions. One common example involves an OCD individual with contamination obsessions and washing compulsions who worries excessively about contracting an illness, germs, and cleanliness. In such cases, the excessive worry contains themes that are obviously related to the individual's obsessions and compulsions, and GAD is easily ruled out. Indeed, no diagnostic disagreements were found when distinguishing OCD from GAD in a large empirical investigation of DSM-IV test-retest diagnostic reliability (Brown, DiNardo, Lehman, & Campbell 2001).

In other cases, however, GAD may be misdiagnosed in place of undetected OCD. More subtle forms of OCD-related worry are sometimes found within the "pure obsessional" OCD subtype. In a recent case study report, Ritter and Hazlett-Stevens (2006) described a client who presented with complaints of excessive and uncontrollable worry about the physical safety of his family. Further questioning revealed recurrent and distressing images, urges, and impulses to harm his family (i.e., obsessions). Not surprisingly, the client was terrified by the content of his unwanted obsessions and was quite reluctant to disclose them at first. Careful assessment also revealed that the client frequently engaged in covert neutralizing responses such as thought suppression, mental distraction, and pleasant imagery replacement (i.e., compulsions). The client and therapist soon discovered that the client's worry about safety also functioned as a covert compulsion. Thus, the anxiety caused by unwanted urges to harm his family was subsequently neutralized with worry about the safety of his family. This worry reassured the client that he really did care about his family and did not secretly wish to hurt them. This case study raised the intriguing possibility that worry may function as a cognitive avoidance response to unwanted obsessions among some OCD individuals. In this case, the excessive and uncontrollable worry and associated generalized anxiety symptoms were considered part of the OCD symptom profile and an additional diagnosis of GAD was not warranted.

Finally, distinguishing GAD from unipolar mood (depressive) disorders is complicated by their considerable symptom overlap. DSM-IV diagnostic criteria for a major depressive episode also include sleep disturbance, fatigue, irritability, restlessness, and difficulty concentrating. Dysthymic disorder is characterized by less severe but more chronic symptoms of sleep disturbance, low energy or fatigue, and poor concentration. If a client experiences these symptoms as part of a major depressive disorder or dysthymic disorder diagnosis, then the clinician must determine whether GAD symptoms only occur during the course of the mood disorder. DSM-IV recognizes excessive worry and generalized anxiety symptoms as common associated features of mood disorders. Therefore, the DSM-IV requires that GAD symptoms are present during a 6-month period in which mood disorder diagnostic criteria have not been met. When a mood disorder exists, a separate GAD diagnosis cannot be made if symptoms occur exclusively during the course of the mood disorder. Clinicians must carefully assess when periods of mood disorder symptoms and GAD symptoms have occurred to determine if an additional GAD diagnosis is appropriate.

## Unstructured Intake Interview Approach

GAD is typically diagnosed following an in-depth clinical interview. A detailed account of the nature and severity of the client's symptoms, associated distress, and functional impairment is collected via open-ended as well as probing follow-up questions. In most clinical practices, this initial diagnostic interview is relatively unstructured. Most clinicians follow a general outline, in which they open with a question about the client's reason for seeking help. The clinician then follows up with more directive questions about the course, history, and frequency of specific symptoms, the impact of symptoms on social and occupational functioning, and the client's subjective experience or conceptualization of these difficulties. Other topics covered in this initial interview include identifiable environmental stressors, medical history, and psychosocial history. During this interview, the clinician also conducts a mental status exam. Observations of the client's appearance, behavior, and mood allow the clinician to evaluate insight, judgment, perception, and general cognitive abilities.

After the clinician gathers this information, the DSM-IV is consulted to determine whether full GAD diagnostic criteria are met. Skilled clinicians are usually able to identify differential diagnostic concerns during the interview and ask pointed questions to address these concerns before ending the interview. This unstructured approach appeals to many clinicians for a number of reasons. First, this format allows clinicians the freedom to focus on any clinical issue believed to be important, regardless of whether or not the issue relates to diagnosis. Second, the conversational, natural discourse found in unstructured interviews may facilitate the establishment of rapport and a strong therapeutic alliance. Finally, because clinicians are not following a set of scripted questions, they are free to ask any clarifying questions needed to determine whether diagnostic criteria are met and to rule out any differential diagnoses. Thus, many clinicians consider this unstructured approach more valid than structured diagnostic interviews containing contrived interview questions.

However, this unstructured interview approach is associated with important disadvantages. Due to the lack of systematic interview questions about additional diagnoses, clinicians may miss important comorbid symptoms altogether if clients fail to mention them. On a related note, diagnostic reliability might be adversely affected by the absence of standardized interview procedures. In other words, two clinicians could obtain different diagnostic pictures of the same client simply because they asked different questions during the interview. This issue is particularly relevant to GAD, often considered the least reliable anxiety disorder diagnosis (see Brown & Barlow 2002 for a review). Finally, less experienced clinicians may encounter considerable difficulty staying on the task of diagnostic assessment. In these instances, the freedom afforded by unstructured interviews could delay the systematic collection of important information and prevent efficient diagnosis and treatment planning.

## Semi-Structured Diagnostic Interviews

Fortunately, an excellent compromise exists between unstructured interviews and fully structured diagnostic interview protocols. Semi-structured clinician-administered interviews contain many open-ended questions, inviting clients to speak freely about their presenting problems and symptoms. Important background information regarding recent environmental stressors, medical history, and psychosocial history also is collected. Unlike unstructured interviews, however, semi-structured interviews contain standardized questions to screen for each diagnosis, followed by specific questions designed to target diagnostic criteria. Detailed questions eliciting information needed to make differential diagnostic decisions are also included. Within this structure, clinicians are free to ask any follow-up questions they deem necessary to gather additional information or to clarify responses to the scripted questions. This hybrid interview approach offers many of the same advantages as the unstructured interview approach while striking an optimal balance between diagnostic reliability and validity.

The Anxiety Disorders Interview Schedule for DSM-IV (ADIS-IV) is the leading semi-structured diagnostic clinical interview for the anxiety disorders. Two versions of the ADIS-IV are available. The Lifetime version (ADIS-IV-L; DiNardo, Brown, & Barlow 1994) assesses for the presence of both current and lifetime disorders, generating a timeline for the onset and remission of each. A nonlifetime (standard) version is also available for settings in which only current diagnoses are needed (ADIS-IV; Brown, DiNardo, & Barlow 1994). Both versions provide for the assessment of GAD and common comorbid conditions, including all anxiety, mood, somatoform, and substance use disorders. Screening questions for other major mental disorders such as psychosis are also included. The ADIS-IV begins with an open-ended question about the reason for seeking help (i.e., presenting problem) and follow-up questions about various life stressors. A series of medical history, psychiatric and psychological treatment history, and family psychiatric history questions are included near the end of the interview. At the conclusion of the interview, the clinician assigns a clinical severity rating ranging from 0 to 8 for each diagnosis detected. A rating of 4 ("definitely disturbing/disabling) or greater is required to warrant a full DSM-IV diagnosis. This clinician severity rating scale reflects the notion that the degree of distress, interference, and functional impairment caused by the symptoms falls along an underlying continuum or dimension. Clinicians have the option of administering the Hamilton Anxiety Rating Scale (HARS; Hamilton 1959) and the Hamilton Rating Scale for Depression (Hamilton

1960), which systematically assess the severity of specific anxiety and depression symptoms. However, concerns about the reliability and discriminant validity of these Hamilton measures have recently been raised (see Roemer, Orsillo, & Barlow 2002 for a review). Both ADIS-IV versions are commercially available through Psychological Corporation/Graywind Publications, and a clinician manual and training video also may be purchased.

In the diagnostic assessment of anxiety disorders, the ADIS-IV interviews are preferred over other semi-structured clinical interviews for a number of reasons. First, pointed questions to help clinicians make differential diagnostic decisions are incorporated throughout each diagnostic section of the ADIS-IV. Additional questions about the nature of associated features and avoidance behaviors aid the clinician in treatment planning. In the GAD section of the ADIS-IV, the clinician determines the degree of excessiveness and uncontrollability for several common worry topics, asks what percentage of the day the client feels worried, assesses for common worry triggers as well as the frequency of unprecipitated worry, and inquires about any avoidance or reassurance behaviors that may function to maintain the worry. A second advantage of the ADIS-IV is the inclusion of the clinician severity rating scale, allowing for a dimensional assessment of the severity for each diagnosis. Thus, sub-clinical conditions are also noted for possible inclusion in the treatment plan. Third, the ADIS-IV is organized into separate modules, allowing the clinician to assess selected diagnoses of interest.

Finally, the ADIS-IV demonstrates strong diagnostic reliability. In a large-scale investigation, Brown et al. (2001) collected data from two independent administrations of the ADIS-IV-L for each of 362 treatment-seeking outpatients. Test-retest diagnostic reliability for each anxiety and unipolar mood disorder was evaluated with a kappa coefficient, providing a more stringent measure of interrater agreement than percent agreement. The kappa coefficient for a current principal GAD diagnosis was 0.67, reflecting a good agreement between independent diagnostic interviewers. Good agreement was also found when GAD was assigned as either a principal or an additional diagnosis (kappa = 0.65). These values demonstrate stronger test-retest reliability for the ADIS-IV-L than the Structured Clinical Interview for DSM-IV Axis I Disorders (SCID-I/P; First, Spitzer, Gibbon, & Williams 2001). In their investigation of DSM-IV diagnostic reliability using the SCID, Zanarini, Skodol, Bender, Dolan, et al. (2000) reported a median kappa of only 0.44 for the diagnosis of GAD. The kappa values reported by Brown et al. (i.e., 0.67 and 0.65) also reflect a substantial improvement in GAD diagnostic reliability when compared to a previous investigation using DSM-III-R diagnostic criteria (kappa=0.57 for principal GAD diagnosis and kappa=0.53 for principal or additional GAD diagnosis; DiNardo, Moras, Barlow, Rapee, & Brown 1993). Improved interrater agreement was also found for many other diagnoses, as kappa coefficients reflecting good to excellent reliability were found for most of the other diagnostic categories examined. In sum, the ADIS-IV-L has strong diagnostic reliability for GAD as well as other anxiety and mood disorders, many of which are common comorbid conditions.

Brown et al. (2001) further examined the factors contributing to interrater disagreements. In the vast majority (74%) of GAD diagnostic disagreement cases, one of the two interviewers assigned a different mood or anxiety disorder diagnosis with similar clinical features. Alternative diagnoses of anxiety disorder not otherwise specified (NOS), dysthymic disorder, and major depressive disorder were the most common. The most frequent sources of diagnostic unreliability identified were differences in patient report, interviewer error, and diagnosis subsumed under a comorbid disorder.

Although the ADIS-IV is typically considered the gold standard in anxiety disorders diagnostic assessment, this interview is quite time-consuming to administer (ranging between 2 and 5 hours) and is limited to certain disorders of interest (anxiety, mood, somatoform, and substance use disorders). Other widely-used semi-structured diagnostic interviews that allow for diagnostic assessment of GAD include the Structured Clinical Interview for DSM-IV Axis I Disorders (SCID-I/P; First et al. 2001) and the Schedule for Affective Disorders and Schizophrenia (SADS-LA-IV; Fyer, Endicott, Mannuza, & Klein 1995). The reader is referred to Summerfeldt and Antony (2002) for a detailed account of these alternative semi-structured diagnostic interviews.

## Structured Diagnostic Interviews

Fully structured diagnostic interviews attempt to remove the need for clinician judgment when making diagnostic decisions. This approach enables lay interviewers to administer diagnostic interviews for the purpose of large-scale epidemiological research. Semi-structured interviews are not completely standardized and allow clinicians to ask follow-up questions to guide diagnostic decision-making. In contrast, the interviewer is afforded no such liberty in the case of fully structured interviews. Each question is read verbatim and can only be repeated, not reworded. Responses are typically recorded according to their forced-choice (i.e., "yes" or "no") format, and a diagnosis results when the right combination of responses are made. Examples of fully structured interviews include the Diagnostic Interview Schedule, Version IV (DIS-IV; Robins, Cottler, Bucholz, & Compton 1995) and the Composite International Diagnostic Interview version 2.1 (CIDI; World Health Organization 1997). Fully structured interviews are needed for research settings in which lay interviewers without clinical training conduct the diagnostic interviews. However, these interviews are rarely used in clinical practice due to concerns about their reliability and validity. For further discussion of fully structured interviews, see Summerfeldt and Antony (2002) and Andrews and Peters (1998).

## Brief Diagnostic Assessment Measures

While comprehensive clinician-administered diagnostic interviews are considered the ideal way to obtain diagnostic information, their administration is not always feasible. Managed care and primary care medical settings often warrant brief diagnostic screening procedures. This issue is particularly relevant to GAD, as GAD individuals often seek treatment from their primary care medical provider (Roy-Byrne & Wagner 2004). Two types of brief diagnostic procedures are available: short clinician-administered interviews and diagnostic screening questionnaires.

The Mini International Neuropsychiatric Interview for DSM-IV, English version 5.0.0 (MINI; Sheehan & Lecrubier 2002) is a clinician-administered structured interview designed to assess most anxiety, mood, eating, substance use, and psychotic disorders. This interview contains very specific close-ended questions, a format which allows administration to take only 15–25 min. Good GAD diagnostic reliability was demonstrated for a previous version of the MINI based on DSM-III-R diagnostic criteria (Sheehan, Lecrubier, Harnett-Sheehan, Janavs, et al. 1997), but no subsequent research has evaluated the psychometric properties of the current DSM-IV version.

The Primary Care Evaluation of Mental Disorders (PRIME-MD; Spitzer, Williams, Kroenke, Linzer, et al. 1994) is a brief semi-structured interview specifically designed for primary care medical practitioners. Primary care patients first complete a brief questionnaire (Patient Health Questionnaire) in which they indicate whether or not they have experienced various DSM-IV psychiatric symptoms. The primary care clinician then administers diagnostic modules of the interview which correspond to those items endorsed on the questionnaire. Using DSM-III-R diagnostic criteria, an initial investigation revealed fair agreement between PRIME-MD diagnosis and diagnosis obtained by an independent mental health professional evaluation among cases of GAD (kappa = 0.52; Spitzer et al. 1994). Diagnostic agreement was good overall (kappa = 0.71; 88% accuracy rate), and primary care physicians completed the interview in an average of 8.4 min. A follow-up study using current DSM-IV criteria reported better GAD diagnostic reliability when clinician-administered PRIME-MD diagnosis was compared to clinician-administered SCID diagnosis (kappa = 0.61; Kobak, Taylor, Dottl, Greist, et al. 1997). However, acceptable GAD diagnostic agreement was not found when a computer-administered telephone interview version of the PRIME-MD was administered instead. Preliminary evidence also supports use of the Patient Health Questionnaire alone as a reliable and valid diagnostic screening measure (Spitzer, Kroenke, & Williams 1999), but diagnostic reliability information specific to GAD was not presented.

Diagnostic screening questionnaires are self-report measures completed by patients, clients, or research participants in the absence of a clinical interview. Such measures are often used in large-scale research projects or survey studies in which administration of individual clinical interviews are not possible. Diagnostic screening questionnaires are also becoming increasingly popular in medical settings; patients who score positive for mental or emotional disorders are referred to appropriate behavioral health providers. Most psychiatric screening instruments measure the degree of psychopathology or psychosocial impairment but do not assess for specific diagnoses. However, the Psychiatric Diagnostic Screening Questionnaire (PDSQ; Zimmerman & Mattia 2001a) reliably assesses DSM-IV diagnostic criteria for 13 different disorders, including GAD. This 126-item measure can be completed in the waiting room within 15–20 min. The original GAD subscale was comprised of five items with adequate internal consistency (Cronbach's alpha = 0.84) and test-retest reliability (correlation coefficient = 0.72; Zimmerman & Mattia 1999). Evidence of strong internal consistency (Cronbach's alpha = 0.89), test-retest reliability (correlation coefficient = 0.79), as well as convergent, concurrent, and discriminant validity was found for the final 10-item GAD subscale (Zimmerman & Mattia 2001a). The 10-item GAD subscale from the final 126-item version of the PDSQ has an associated sensitivity of 90% and specificity of 50% (Zimmerman & Mattia 2001b).

Another diagnostic screening questionnaire was specifically designed to identify individuals with GAD. The Generalized Anxiety Disorder Questionnaire-IV (GAD-Q-IV; Newman, Zuellig, Kachin, Constantino, et al. 2002) is based on the original GAD-Q (Roemer, Borkovec, Posa, & Borkovec 1995), a single-page pencil-and-paper measure developed to detect the presence of GAD diagnosis. Revised to reflect current DSM-IV diagnostic criteria, the GAD-Q-IV contains checklists for required symptoms as well as Likert rating scales to assess degree of interference and distress resulting from worry and associated symptoms. A total score is calculated according to a scoring system, and GAD is detected when this total score falls above a designated cutoff score. This GAD-Q-IV scoring system yielded 89% specificity and 83% sensitivity in initial Receiver Operating Characteristics analyses (Newman et al. 2002). Strong test-retest reliability (kappa = 0.64) and convergent and discriminant validity were also demonstrated. Finally, Newman and colleagues reported a kappa coefficient of 0.67 when GAD diagnosis obtained with the GAD-Q-IV was compared to results from an independent administration of the ADIS-IV clinical interview. However, subsequent research with ethnically diverse samples suggested that the GAD-Q-IV might over-diagnose GAD when the dimensional scoring system is used (Roemer, Salters, Raffa, & Orsillo 2005; Turk, Heimberg, Luterek, Mennin, & Fresco 2005). Matching item responses to the respective DSM-IV diagnostic criteria appeared to address this problem (Turk et al.). In sum, the GAD-Q-IV is a brief self-report instrument that reliably identified individuals with GAD and distinguished GAD individuals from social phobia, panic disorder, and nonanxious control participants (Newman et al. 2002). Importantly, the diagnostic reliability of the GAD-Q-IV was comparable to that obtained for clinician-administered ADIS-IV interviews. Newman and colleagues recommended that clinicians and researchers use the GAD-Q-IV as an initial screening device, followed by an in-depth clinical interview.

## *Summary and Conclusions*

Diagnostic assessment procedures allow clinicians to evaluate specific GAD symptoms and to establish whether diagnostic criteria have been met. Clinicians also must determine whether symptoms can be better accounted for by another diagnosis, as excessive worry is often seen in other psychological disorders. GAD should not be diagnosed if symptoms occur exclusively during the course of a mood disorder. Diagnostic assessment typically begins with a clinician-administered interview. Although unstructured diagnostic interviews are common to private practice settings, semi-structured diagnostic interviews offer several advantages. Like unstructured interviews, semi-structured interviews include open-ended questions and allow clinicians the freedom to ask any follow-up questions they deem necessary. However, semi-structured interviews also contain specific questions that aid clinicians in making differential diagnostic decisions. In addition, semi-structured interviews assess comorbid conditions that might not be revealed during the course of an unstructured interview. The ADIS-IV is the leading semi-structured interview for use with anxiety disorder clinical populations. Brief diagnostic assessment procedures, including short clinician-administered interviews and screening questionnaires, are also available. These alternative procedures can be useful in settings where time-consuming diagnostic clinical interviews are not feasible.

Many mental health clinicians may benefit from a careful examination of their own diagnostic assessment procedures. Practitioners who rely on unstructured intake interviews alone to gather initial diagnostic information might consider incorporating other procedures into their clinical evaluations. For example, clients could complete a diagnostic screening questionnaire, such as the PHQ from the PRIME-MD, the PDSQ, or the GAD-Q-IV, in the waiting room before an initial appointment. Their responses could guide clinicians in selecting relevant ADIS-IV modules to administer during the consultation process. Accurate diagnosis is an important first step in treatment planning, as most empirically-supported treatments were developed for specific diagnostic groups. Nevertheless, clients who do not meet full GAD diagnostic criteria or do not receive a GAD diagnosis because their symptoms coincide with a mood disorder still may benefit from the treatment approach described in this book. Additional measures useful in the assessment of GAD and chronically worried individuals are described next.

## Assessment of Worry and Related Constructs

Many standardized self-report instruments assess anxiety, stress, and negative affectivity. However, most do not target GAD-specific constructs and therefore cannot distinguish GAD from other anxiety disorders. These self-report questionnaires measure the tendency to experience anxiety, severity of anxiety symptoms, and associated negative affect or distress. Similar to the clinician-administered Hamilton Anxiety Rating Scale (HARS; Hamilton 1959), such measures capture the symptoms, complaints, and experiences of anxiety disorder clients but do not shed light on the underlying cognitive and affective factors believed to maintain GAD. Popular examples include the State-Trait Anxiety Inventory (STAI; Spielberger, Gorsuch, Lushene, Vagg, & Jacobs 1983), the Depression Anxiety Stress Scales (DASS; Lovibond & Lovibond 1995), the Mood and Anxiety Symptoms Questionnaire (MASQ; Watson, Weber, Assenheimer, Clark, et al. 1995) and the Trimodal Anxiety Questionnaire

(TAQ; Lehrer & Woolfolk 1982). The well-known Beck Anxiety Inventory (BAI; Beck & Steer 1990) and Beck Depression Inventory (BDI; Beck & Steer 1987) also assess common anxiety and depression symptoms, although the BAI measures autonomic hyperarousal rather than the central nervous system somatic symptoms typical of GAD. General measures of an individual's tendency to experience negative emotions and affect include the Positive and Negative Affect Scales (PANAS; Watson, Clark, & Tellegen 1988), the Neuroticism subscales of the Eysenck Personality Questionnaire (EPQ; Eysenck & Eysenck 1975) and the NEO-PI-R (Costa & McCrae 1992), and the Behavioral Inhibition System Sensitivity Scale from the BIS/BAS Scales (Carver & White 1994). Further information about these and other anxiety measures can be found in Roemer (2001a).

Personality inventories such as the Minnesota Multiphasic Personality Inventory-2 (MMPI-2) and the Millon Clinical Multiaxial Inventory (MCMI-III) also contain scales that reflect neurotic personality traits and anxiety symptoms. For example, GAD individuals are expected to show elevations (i.e., above the clinical cutoff T-score of 65) on the MMPI-2 clinical scale 7 ("Psychasthenia"), reflecting the degree to which individuals tend to feel anxious, tense, worried, and apprehensive (Graham 2006). Elevated scale 7 scores also are expected for individuals with other anxiety disorders, particularly OCD. This scale reflects degree of psychological distress and a tendency toward anxiety-related symptoms and experiences but is not useful in discriminating GAD from other anxiety disorders. Similar claims have been made about the MMPI-2 content and supplementary Anxiety scales (ANX and A, respectively; see Graham 2006), as well as the Anxiety (A) clinical syndrome scale of the MCMI-III. Like the questionnaire measures listed above, individuals with GAD are expected to exhibit clinical elevations on these scales but such test results do not aid in making differential diagnosis decisions. Furthermore, none of these scales reflect constructs specifically implicated in the etiology and maintenance of GAD. These anxiety and personality measures are useful in detecting the presence of clinical anxiety, assessing the severity of various symptoms, and measuring general personality traits seen in anxious individuals. A different array of self-report measures targeting the chronic worry and cognitive features central to GAD are reviewed in this section. Many of these measures are reprinted in the *Practitioner's Guide to Empirically Based Measures of Anxiety* edited by Antony, Orsillo, and Roemer (2001).

## Worry Severity

The Penn State Worry Questionnaire (PSWQ; Meyer, Miller, Metzger, & Borkovec 1990) is a widely-used measure of chronic worry. The PSWQ contains 16 items designed to assess excessiveness, uncontrollability, and severity of an individual's worry. Five of these items are reverse-scored and ask about the degree to which worry is absent. None of the PSWQ items reflect specific worry content. Thus, the PSWQ was developed as a measure of worry frequency and severity without focus on specific worry domains. Examples of items include "My worries overwhelm me" and "Once I start worrying, I can't stop." Respondents rate the extent to which each item is typical of them on a 5-point Likert scale (1 = "Not at all typical," 3 = "Somewhat typical," 5 = "Very typical"). A total score is computed by reversing the ratings on the five reverse-scored items (i.e., 1 = 5, 2 = 4, 4 = 2, 5 = 1) and then summing up all item ratings. Possible total scores therefore range from 16 to 80, with higher scores reflecting higher levels of trait worry.

Average scores tend to fall around the middle of the scale. For example, the mean PSWQ score reported for unselected college student samples was 47.65 ($SD$ = 12.99) (Molina & Borkovec 1994) and a 50th percentile PSWQ score of 41 was reported for a normative community sample (Gillis, Haaga, & Ford 1995). Treatment-seeking clients diagnosed with GAD scored a mean of 67.66 ($SD$ = 8.86) on the PSWQ, and college students endorsing full DSM-III-R GAD diagnostic criteria on the original GAD-Q scored an average of 63.24 ($SD$ = 9.33) (Molina & Borkovec 1994). Receiver operating characteristics (ROC) analysis investigations demonstrated that a PSWQ cutoff score of 62 identified cases of GAD (using DSM-IV criteria) with an optimal balance between sensitivity and specificity, effectively discriminating GAD from PTSD and depression (Behar, Alcaine, Zuellig, & Borkovec 2003). This cutoff score was not as useful when discriminating between GAD and social phobia, and a follow-up ROC investigation found that a PSWQ cutoff score of 65 better identified GAD relative to social phobia individuals (Fresco, Mennin, Heimberg, & Turk 2003).

While GAD individuals are indeed elevated on the PSWQ, this measure also identifies individuals reporting excessive and uncontrollable worry who do not meet DSM-IV diagnostic criteria for GAD. A PSWQ score of 51 fell at the 80th percentile in the normative community sample study (Gillis et al. 1995). In addition, Ruscio (2002) found that 28% of a college sample scored at or above a PSWQ cutoff score of 56, a score falling one standard deviation below the reported mean for GAD individuals diagnosed following ADIS-IV administration. Ruscio concluded that a substantial portion of college students may suffer from severe and frequent worry, although only 6% reported full GAD diagnostic criteria on the GAD-Q-IV. Individuals scoring above this 56 cutoff who did not meet GAD diagnostic criteria did endorse associated anxiety symptoms, distress, and functional impairment to some degree. Individuals reporting excessive and uncontrollable chronic worry by scoring 56 or higher on the PSWQ therefore may benefit from the treatment approach described in this book even if full GAD diagnostic criteria are not met.

Research investigations consistently report strong internal consistency for the PSWQ with alpha coefficients ranging from 0.86 to 0.93 (Molina & Borkovec 1994). Reported test-retest reliability correlation coefficients range from 0.74 to 0.93 (Molina & Borkovec), suggesting that PSWQ trait worry scores are stable over time. Many studies also support the validity of the PSWQ (see Turk, Heimberg, & Mennin 2004 for a review), and GAD individuals scored higher on the PSWQ than individuals with other anxiety disorder diagnoses (Brown, Antony, & Barlow 1992). The PSWQ was originally developed as a unifactorial scale, with all items selected to measure the single construct of pathological worry (Meyer et al. 1990). However, subsequent factor analysis research found that the five reverse-scored items loaded on a separate factor (e.g., Fresco, Heimberg, Mennin, & Turk 2002). Other researchers have found that the one-factor model indeed provided the best fit to the data once method-factor variance was taken into account (Brown 2003; Hazlett-Stevens, Ullman, & Craske 2004).

In sum, the PSWQ is an excellent and well-established measure of problematic worry. PSWQ cutoff scores ranging from 62 to 65 distinguish GAD from other anxiety disorder individuals. The PSWQ may also identify clients who struggle with chronic worry in the absence of a GAD diagnosis; a cutoff score of 56 has been recommended for this purpose. This pencil-and-paper measure can be completed within 2–3 min in the waiting room to screen for excessive and uncontrollable worry. Although the original PSWQ was designed as a stable measure of trait worry, a Past-Week version can be used to monitor progress in treatment (PSWQ-PW; Stöber & Bittencourt 1998).

## *Worry Content*

The Worry Domains Questionnaire (WDQ; Tallis, Eysenck, & Mathews 1992) measures the overall degree to which an individual worries as well as the amount of worry in each of five specific content areas, or domains: (1) Relationships, (2) Lack of Confidence, (3) Aimless Future, (4) Work, and (5) Financial. Individuals respond to each of the 25 WDQ items by indicating the degree to which they worry about that specific topic on a 5-point Likert scale (0 = "Not at all," 1 = "A little," 2 = "Moderately," 3 = "Quite a bit," 4 = "Extremely"). A total score is calculated by summing all item scores for use as a general measure of worry. Then separate domain scores are calculated by summing the items contained in each domain. For example, Relationships domain items include "that I find it difficult to maintain a stable relationship" and "that I am unattractive." Lack of Confidence items include "that I feel insecure," aimless future items include "that I'll never achieve my ambitions," Work items include "that I will not keep my workload up to date," and Financial items include "that my money will run out."

The WDQ was originally developed to measure normal worry among non-clinical individuals for research purposes. However, this questionnaire might be added to the PSWQ in clinical settings to identify topic areas of greatest concern. The mean WDQ total score reported for a treatment-seeking GAD clinical sample was 40.03 (*SD* = 19.8), compared to an employed community sample mean of 23.1 (*SD* = 13.4) and a college student mean of 26.6 (13.0) (Tallis, Davey, & Bond 1994). Interestingly, a comparison OCD clinical sample scored a mean of 50.07 (20.8). Individual domain scale means and standard deviations for each of these samples were also reported by Tallis and colleagues. For the clinical GAD group, the following means and standard deviations were found: Relationships: 5.7 (5.6); Lack of Confidence: 10.2 (4.7); Aimless Future: 9.5 (5.1); Work: 7.7 (4.5); Financial: 7.1

(5.0). GAD individuals scored higher on the WDQ than nonanxious individuals, and GAD individuals also scored higher on the WDQ than individuals with other anxiety disorders (Ladouceur, Dugas, Freeston, Rhéaume, et al. 1999). However, as mentioned above, the WDQ might not be useful distinguishing GAD from OCD (Tallis et al. 1994).

Not surprisingly, the domain subscale scores were significantly correlated with each other ($r$'s ranging from 0.24 to 0.66; Tallis et al. 1994), and WDQ total scores correlated with other worry and anxiety measures, such as the PSWQ ($r = 0.67$; Tallis et al.). Results from several investigations provided evidence of good internal consistency, test-retest reliability, and validity of the WDQ (see Turk et al. 2004 for a review). One large confirmatory factor analysis investigation supported the factor structure of the original WDQ (Joormann & Stöber 1997). However, a similar investigation found that some WDQ items did not load highest on their respective domain subscale factors (Van Rijsoort, Emmelkamp, & Vervaeke 1999). These authors revised the WDQ by reassigning items according to factor analysis results and expanded the original WDQ by adding 5 items tapping the domain of health worry (WDQ-R; Van Rijsoort et al. 1999). While both versions of the WDQ were most often studied among non-clinical populations, either one might be useful in clinical settings to assess the degree to which clients worry about a variety of topic areas. Inspection of individual item scores may alert the clinician to specific concerns most salient for a given client.

## Meta-Worry

The Anxious Thoughts Inventory (AnTI; Wells 1994) measures worry about the specific topics of social interaction and physical health. In addition, a meta-worry subscale assesses worry about the negative consequences of worry itself. The AnTI includes 22 items and measures the degree to which an individual worries about three separate areas: social worry, health worry, and meta-worry. Respondents rate how frequently they worry about the topic reflected in each item using a 4-point Likert scale (1 = "Almost never," 4 = "Almost always"). Examples of items include "I worry about my appearance" (social), "I worry about death" (health), and "I think that I am missing out on things in life because I worry too much" (meta-worry).

Reported means for GAD individuals on the separate AnTI subscales were 24.0 ($SD = 5.1$) for social worry, 14.3 ($SD = 3.6$) for health worry, and 19.7 ($SD = 3.9$) for meta-worry (Wells & Carter 2001). Means obtained from an unselected community control sample were 17.5 ($SD = 4.6$) for social worry, 10.0 ($SD = 3.3$) for health worry, and 12.8 ($SD = 3.8$) for meta-worry, all of which were significantly lower than the GAD group means. The third subscale, meta-worry, has generated the most research interest, as this particular construct has been implicated in the development of GAD (Wells 2004). The social worry and health worry subscales were designed to measure normal worry processes, whereas the meta-worry subscale was developed to measure a pathological process leading to GAD. Accordingly, Wells and Carter (1999) found that only the meta-worry subscale predicted PSWQ scores; social and health worry subscale AnTI scores did not. The meta-worry subscale also distinguished GAD individuals from panic disorder, social phobia, and control group individuals (Wells & Carter 2001). Wells (1994) demonstrated acceptable internal consistency for each subscale (social worry alpha coefficient = 0.84; health worry alpha coefficient = 0.81; meta-worry alpha coefficient = 0.75) as well as test-retest reliability ($r$'s ranging from 0.76 to 0.84). In short, the AnTI might be a useful pencil-and paper measure for clients reporting excessive worry about social and/or health concerns as well as worry about worry itself (i.e., meta-worry).

Wells recently published an expanded measure of meta-worry, the Meta-worry Questionnaire (MWQ; Wells 2005). Seven items reflecting major meta-worry themes derived from GAD treatment sessions were constructed. Respondents rated each item on two different response scales: frequency of that meta-worry and the degree of belief in that meta-worry at the time of its occurrence. The frequency scale utilized a 4-point Likert scale response format (1 = "Never," 2 = "Sometimes," 3 = "Often," 4 = "Always"), and the belief scale responses ranged from 0 to 100 (0 = I do not believe this thought at all and 100 = I am completely convinced this thought is true). Although scale scores were not normally distributed, Wells found evidence of good internal reliability and validity. Factor analysis results suggested a single factor structure underlying each scale. As predicted, GAD individuals scored higher on the MWQ frequency scale than somatic anxiety and nonanxious control groups. GAD individuals also scored higher on the MWQ belief scale than nonanxious individuals. Importantly, these group differences remained after statistically controlling for AnTI social worry and health worry subscale scores. Thus, the meta-worry themes contained in the MWQ may detect GAD better than the AnTI worry domain subscales.

## *Worry Beliefs*

A few measures assess beliefs about the benefits of worry, as many GAD clients endorse positive beliefs about their worry despite its accompanying negative effects (e.g., Borkovec, Hazlett-Stevens, & Diaz 1999). A brief six-item questionnaire named the Reasons To Worry Questionnaire (Borkovec & Roemer 1995) was developed to examine whether GAD and nonanxious individuals endorsed different perceived functions of their worry. Respondents rated the degree to which each of the six statements represented a reason for their worry using a 1- to 5-point Likert scale (1 = "Not at all," 5 = "Very much"). Each item was written to reflect a different reason for worry, such as motivation, problem-solving, preparation, prevention, and superstition. Borkovec and Roemer found that GAD individuals endorsed worry as a distraction from even more emotional topics the individual does not want to think about more than nonanxious individuals did. This finding was replicated in a second sample. Psychometric data for this brief measure are not available. Nevertheless, clinicians might initiate fruitful discussions with their GAD clients by exploring each of the statements contained in this measure.

The Why Worry? Scale (WW; Freeston, Rhéaume, Letarte, Dugas, & Ladouceur 1994) and the updated Why Worry-II Scale (reprinted in Antony, Orsillo, & Roemer 2001) provide psychometrically sound measures of positive worry beliefs. The original WW measure contained 20 items, each stating a perceived benefit of worry. Respondents rate how true each worry belief is for them on a 5-point Likert scale (1 = "Not at all true," 2 = "Slightly true," 3 = "Somewhat true," 4 = "Very true," 5 = "Absolutely true"). The revised 25-item WW-II is comprised of five subscales, each containing five items reflecting the different types of perceived worry benefits: worry aids in problem-solving ("I worry in order to know what to do"), worry helps to motivate ("The fact that I worry incites me to act"), worrying protects from negative emotions ("If I worry in advance, I will be less disappointed if something serious occurs"), worrying prevents negative outcomes ("The act of worrying itself can prevent mishaps from occurring"), and worry is a positive personality trait ("If I did not worry, I would be careless and irresponsible").

High internal consistency and convergent validity have been demonstrated for both the WW and WW-II (see Roemer 2001b for a review). Although WW mean scores have been reported for college student and GAD samples (Freeston et al. 1994; Ladouceur, Blais, Freeston, & Dugas 1998), normative data are not currently available for the revised WW-II. However, the WW-II subscales may also aid clinicians in identifying clients' specific beliefs about why they need to worry.

A final worry beliefs questionnaire measures both negative and positive beliefs about worry: the Consequences of Worry Scale (COWS; Davey, Tallis, & Capuzzo 1996). For each of the 29 items, respondents rate how much they believe that consequence describes their worry on a 5-point Likert scale (1 = "Not at all," 2 = "A little," 3 = "Moderately," 4 = "Quite a bit," 5 = "A lot"). Total negative consequences and total positive consequences scores are calculated. In addition, three negative consequences subscales include disrupting performance ("When I worry, it stops me from taking decisive action"), exaggerating the problem ("Problems are magnified when I dwell on them"), and causing emotional distress ("Worrying makes me tense and irritable"). The two positive consequences subscales include motivational influence ("In order to get something done, I have to worry about it"), and helping analytical thinking ("Worrying gives me the opportunity to analyze situations and work out the pros and cons").

Although research has demonstrated convergent validity and acceptable internal consistency for each subscale of the COWS (alpha coefficients range from 0.72 to 0.87; Davey et al. 1996), only unselected college student samples were studied. Unfortunately, clinical sample and normative data are not available for this measure. Nevertheless, inspection of the individual items might help clinicians identify clients' strongest worry beliefs. Davey and colleagues found that college students endorsing a combination of positive and negative worry beliefs scored higher on psychopathology measures than students endorsing only negative beliefs about the consequences of worry.

Worry beliefs are traditionally assessed with the self-report questionnaires described above. However, Francis and Dugas (2004) have recently developed a structured interview for this purpose. The Structured Interview on Beliefs About Worry (SIBAW; Francis & Dugas 2004) contains four subscales, each reflecting a different positive worry belief: (1) worry aids problem-solving and motivation, (2) worry protects from negative emotions, (3) worry as a positive personality trait, and (4) worry as a mental act can directly alter events (i.e., magical thinking). After a "target worry" is selected, each interview subscale begins with an unscored open question introducing the content of that subscale worry belief. Next, a series of specific scored items are presented in which clients rate their endorsement of each on a 9-point Likert scale (0 – "Not at all" and 8 = "Completely"). Although normative data are not yet available, initial research identified the four-factor structure and provided evidence of high internal consistency and good validity and test-retest reliability (Francis & Dugas 2004). This promising new instrument may allow for a comprehensive assessment of worry beliefs to be incorporated into other clinical interview protocols.

## Other Meta-Cognitive Constructs

Other self-report instruments assess beliefs about intrusive thoughts and cognitive processes more generally. These questionnaires may reveal underlying beliefs that unwanted thoughts are inherently harmful and should be avoided or controlled. Similar to worry beliefs, other meta-cognitive beliefs and thought control strategies could potentially undermine therapeutic interventions unless directly addressed. The Meta-Cognitions Questionnaire (MCQ; Cartwright-Hatton & Wells 1997) is a 65-item measure of positive and negative worry beliefs as well as lack of confidence in cognitive processes and the degree to which an individual monitors such thought processes. Respondents rate how much they agree with each item statement using a 4-point Likert scale (1 = "Do not agree," 2 = "Agree slightly," 3 = "Agree moderately," 4 = "Agree very much"). Five subscale scores are calculated by reverse-scoring items worded in the opposite direction and then summing the item scores that comprise each subscale. The separate factor-analytically derived subscales are: Positive Worry Beliefs ("Worrying helps me to avoid problems in the future"), Beliefs about Controllability and Danger ("I could make myself sick with worrying"), Beliefs about Cognitive Competence ("I have little confidence in my memory for words and names"), General Negative Beliefs ("I could be punished for not having certain thoughts"), and Cognitive Self-consciousness ("I think a lot about my thoughts").

Cartwright-Hatton and Wells (1997) reported the following MCQ subscale means for GAD individuals: Positive Beliefs, 32.9 ($SD$ = 10.0); Uncontrollability and Danger, 47.5 ($SD$ = 7.7), Cognitive Competence, 22.8 ($SD$ = 8.0); General

Negative Beliefs, 27.7 (*SD* = 6.2); Cognitive Self-consciousness, 16.5 (*SD* = 5.4). Subscale means reported for a nonanxious control sample were: Positive Beliefs, 29.6 (*SD* = 8.8); Uncontrollability and Danger, 26.0 (*SD* = 6.3), Cognitive Competence, 15.5 (*SD* = 4.2); General Negative Beliefs, 19.7 (*SD* = 6.4); Cognitive Self-consciousness, 14.9 (*SD* = 4.1).

Adequate internal consistency (alpha coefficients ranged from 0.72 to 0.89), test-retest reliability (*r*'s ranged from 0.76 to 0.89), and validity were demonstrated for the MCQ subscales (Cartwright-Hatton & Wells 1997). Consistent with their meta-cognitive theory of GAD, Wells and Carter (2001) found that GAD individuals scored significantly higher on both negative worry belief scales (Uncontrollability and Danger and General Negative Beliefs) than a community control sample as well as social phobia and panic disorder clinical samples. College students endorsing GAD diagnostic criteria on the original GAD-Q scored higher than nonanxious students on all MCQ subscales, although no differences were found between the GAD group and a nonworried anxious comparison group on the Positive Beliefs subscale (Davis & Valentiner 2000). Thus, the MCQ is a useful measure of various meta-cognitive beliefs, and the Uncontrollability and Danger and the General Negative Beliefs subscales in particular appear to discriminate GAD from social phobia and panic disorder.

The specific meta-cognitive belief that thinking certain thoughts actually increases the likelihood of unwanted events can also be measured. The Thought-Action Fusion scale (TAF; Shafran, Thordarson, & Rachman 1996) contains two "Likelihood" subscales targeting these particular superstitious beliefs. Originally developed to measure the magical thinking component observed in OCD, the TAF contains three subscales: (1) Likelihood-for-self, or the degree to which thoughts are believed to affect the likelihood of unwanted events happening to oneself, (2) Likelihood-for-others, or the degree to which thoughts are believed to affect the likelihood of unwanted events happening to others, and (3) Moral, the degree to which having sinful or immoral thoughts is considered just as immoral as committing such actions. Respondents rate each of the 19 items on a 5-point Likert scale (0 = "Disagree strongly" and 4 = "Agree strongly"). Sharfan and colleagues demonstrated good reliability and validity for each of the three subscales, although the Likelihood-for-others and Likelihood-for-self subscales contain only four and three items, respectively. Administration of the TAF might help clinicians identify specific magical thinking cognitive beliefs about worry and other anxious thoughts. Indeed, Hazlett-Stevens, Zucker, and Craske (2002) found that PSWQ worry scores correlated with both Likelihood TAF subscales and that individuals endorsing GAD diagnostic criteria scored higher on these subscales than nonanxious individuals. However, only PSWQ scores predicted GAD diagnostic status when Likelihood subscale scores and PSWQ scores were entered as predictor variables in a logistic regression analysis. Therefore, while elevated TAF Likelihood beliefs may be explained by excessive and controllable worry among GAD individuals, assessment of these beliefs would allow for them to be explored and challenged in treatment.

The Thought Control Questionnaire (TCQ; Wells & Davies 1994; Wells 2000) is a 30-item scale designed to measure ways in which individuals attempt to control unwanted cognitive activity. Respondents indicate on a 4-point Likert scale (1 = "Never," 2 = "Sometimes," 3 = "Often," 4 = "Almost always") how often they use the technique described in each item when an unpleasant/unwanted thought is experienced. The TCQ is comprised of five subscales, each reflecting a different thought control strategy: Distraction ("I occupy myself with work instead"), Social Control ("I don't talk about the thought to anyone"), Worry ("I worry about more minor things instead"), Punishment ("I tell myself not to be so stupid"), and Re-appraisal ("I challenge the thought's validity"). After reverse-scoring certain items, subscale scores are calculated by summing the item scores for each. A total score can also be calculated to reflect the overall degree of attempted thought control.

Means and standard deviations for the TCQ subscales were reported for a large non-clinical sample using a previous 36-item version (Wells & Davies 1994). Wells (2000) reported the following means for a small (n = 20) GAD clinical sample using the current 30-item version: Distraction, 13.1 (SD = 3.4); Social control, 10.6 (SD = 3.0); Worry, 11.7 (SD = 3.5); Punishment, 13.3 (SD = 3.3); Re-appraisal, 11.3 (SD = 4.0). Descriptive data from panic disorder, major depressive disorder, and PTSD clinical groups were also reported. Descriptive TCQ subscale data are also available for OCD (Amir, Cashman, & Foa 1997) and acute stress disorder (Warda & Bryant 1998) clinical groups. These various clinical groups scored higher on the Worry and Punishment TCQ subscales than control groups. Although reliance on maladaptive thought control strategies is observed across various anxiety and depressive disorders, the TCQ may provide insight into GAD clients' preferred thought control strategies. Of particular interest, scores on the Worry subscale reflect the degree to which clients rely upon worry as a strategy to control other unwanted thoughts.

One final self-report measure of this nature is the Cognitive Avoidance Questionnaire (CAQ; Gosselin, Langlois, Freeston, Ladouceur, et al. 2002). This questionnaire was originally published in French, but an English translation since has become available (Sexton & Dugas 2008). The CAQ assesses the tendency to engage in five cognitive avoidance strategies: suppressing worrisome thoughts, substituting neutral or positive thoughts for worries, distraction to interrupt worrying, avoiding behavior or situations that can lead to worry, and transforming mental images into verbal-linguistic thoughts. A total of 25 items are rated on a 5-point Likert scale, ranging from "not at all characteristic of me" to "entirely characteristic of me." While this questionnaire measure has demonstrated good internal consistency (alpha coefficient of 0.95) and test-retest reliability 4–6 weeks later (r = 0.85), this newer measure has not been examined among clinical samples yet.

## Intolerance of Uncertainty

The Intolerance of Uncertainty Scale (IUS; Freeston et al. 1994) was developed to test the authors' theory that a difficulty tolerating life's uncertainties underlies GAD. Respondents indicate how characteristic each of the 27 items are of them using a 5-point Likert scale (1 = "Not at all," 2 = "A little," 3 = "Somewhat," 4 = "Very,"

5 = "Entirely characteristic of me"). Examples of items include "Uncertainty makes life intolerable," "I always want to know what the future has in store for me," and "The ambiguities in life stress me." The IUS is scored by summing responses to all items, resulting in a total score ranging from 27 to 135.

   Treatment-seeking clients diagnosed with GAD scored an average of 87.08 ($SD$ = 21.08) on the IUS (Ladouceur et al. 2000), whereas the mean reported for a nonanxious college sample was only 43.8 (SD = 10.8) (Freeston et al. 1994). Excellent internal consistency, adequate test-retest reliability, and convergent validity have been demonstrated for the IUS (see Roemer 2001b for a review). In addition, the IUS discriminated GAD individuals from those with other anxiety disorders (Ladouceur, Dugas, Freeston, Rhéaume, et al. 1999) and from nonanxious individuals (Dugas, Gagnon, Ladouceur, & Freeston 1998). The IUS correlated more strongly with the PSWQ than with the Padua Inventory, a measure of obsessive/compulsive symptoms, and the Body Sensations Questionnaire, a measure of panic sensations (Dugas, Gosselin, & Ladouceur 2001). In sum, the IUS is unique in its ability to measure clients' responses to uncertain situations, a factor that appears more central to GAD than the other anxiety disorders. This measure may also be useful for monitoring client progress, as IUS scores significantly decreased following cognitive-behavioral therapy for GAD (Ladouceur et al. 2000).

## *Summary and Conclusions*

Many self-report questionnaires and psychological tests assess common anxiety symptoms and general tendencies toward anxious experience. While these scales provide useful measures of symptom severity, distress, and underlying neurotic traits, they do not differentiate GAD from other anxiety disorders. Furthermore, such measures were not designed to target the specific clinical features and constructs central to GAD. Self-report measures of worry severity, worry content, and meta-worry provide clinicians with crucial information about the nature of an individual's worry process. In addition, assessment of meta-cognitive worry beliefs, thought control strategies, and intolerance of uncertainty can help clinicians identify underlying cognitive processes maintaining excessive worry. Rather than asking clients to complete all of these measures in one sitting, clinicians can selectively administer measures as additional information appears needed for treatment planning. For example, initial diagnostic impressions suggesting the presence of chronic worry could be followed up with the PSWQ. If the PSWQ total score is elevated, administration of worry domain measures, such as the WDQ or AnTI, could reveal which worry topics are of greatest concern to the client. Clients expressing reluctance to reduce worry or who feel that they must worry to cope with life's challenges could be administered worry beliefs and/or other meta-cognitive measures once these issues arise in the course of treatment. With the exception of the SIBAW clinician administered interview (Francis & Dugas 2004) these measures are brief self-report inventories that clients easily could complete in the waiting room before a treatment session.

# Assessment of Older Adults

In their recent review of the literature, Beck and Averill (2004) identified two strategies used to evaluate assessment measures for older adults. One method involves examining the psychometric properties of existing instruments among older adult samples. The second strategy involves developing new measures specifically for use with elderly individuals. Investigations of existing diagnostic interview procedures as well as other measures of anxiety and worry have been conducted with this particular population. In addition, a few measures developed specifically for use with older adults have emerged in the literature.

## *Examination of Existing Measures*

Among available clinician-administered diagnostic measures, Beck and Averill (2004) concluded that previous versions of the ADIS (ADIS-R; DiNardo, Moras, Barlow, Rapee, & Brown 1993) and the SCID (Spitzer, Williams, Gibbon, & First 1988) were potentially useful diagnostic interviews for the assessment of older adults. Beck and Averill cautioned against use of the DIS when working with this population. However, current versions of these instruments based on DSM-IV criteria have not been examined in this regard yet. The clinician-administered Hamilton Anxiety Rating Scale (HARS) provided at the end of the ADIS yielded internally consistent scores among older adults and correctly classified 90% of participants into GAD and control participants groups (Beck, Stanley, & Zebb 1999). However, the HARS may not differentiate anxiety from depression symptoms among older adults. Of the worry-related self-report measures described above, the PSWQ has been studied among elderly samples the most. Among older adults, the PSWQ yielded good internal consistency and adequate convergent validity (Beck, Stanley, & Zebb 1995) but may not be stable over time (Stanley, Novy, Bourland, Beck, & Averill 2001).

## *Assessment Measures Developed for Older Adults*

In the second approach to assessment of older adults identified by Beck and Averill (2004), new measures for specific use with this particular population are developed. A brief clinical interview designed to screen for anxiety symptoms among older clients known as the Short Anxiety Screening Test (SAST; Sinoff, Ore, Zlotogorsky, & Tamir 1999) yielded acceptable levels of sensitivity (75%) and specificity (79%). In addition, two self-report worry measures have been developed specifically for older individuals. The original Worry Scale for Older Adults (WS; Wisocki, Handen, & Morse 1986) contained 35 items to assess degree of worry in social, financial, and health content areas. Each item describes a worry topic, followed by a 5-point Likert scale ranging from "never" to "much of the time." Participants respond to each item by indicating how much they worry about that topic. Means and standard deviations for total scores as well as for each subscale are available for older individuals with GAD and for non-anxious control participants (Stanley, Beck, & Zebb 1996). Evidence of convergent validity and adequate to excellent levels of internal consistency were obtained from total scores and from subscale scores in each sample as well. The original WS was revised and expanded (WSOA-R; Hunt, Wisocki, & Yanko 2003) containing 88 items covering six content areas: finances, health, social conditions, personal concerns, family concerns, and world issues. A separate coping inventory assessing which strategies individuals use to control worry is also available. Psychometric research on the newer WSOA-R found evidence of high internal consistency among older adults (alpha coefficient of 0.97 for total scores and alpha coefficients ranged from 0.88 to 0.95 for the six subscales) and of convergent validity, supported by a significant correlation between WSOA-R and the PSWQ total scores ($r = 0.45$). When compared to a younger adult college student sample, older adults scored higher on the individual subscales of health, family concerns, and world issues.

A second self-report worry measure was developed specifically for older adults residing in nursing homes. The Worry Questionnaire for Nursing Home Residents (WQNHR; Hertzsprung, Konnert, & Brinker 2004) is a brief 15-item measure. Residents indicate how often they worry about specific concerns, some of which are unique to the nursing home environment (e.g., "Your relationships with staff members," "Having to be cared for by people other than your loved ones"). A collateral form (WQNHR-C) was developed for administration to family or friends, but this form did not correlate with WQNHR scores. Preliminary psychometric evaluation yielded adequate internal consistency (alpha coefficient of 0.79), test-retest reliability, and good convergent validity. However, neither the Worry Scale nor the WQNHR appear to discriminate worry from depression.

## Treatment Planning

Comprehensive assessments allow clinicians to construct thoughtful treatment plans. Detailed client-specific information is necessary to develop an effective individually tailored plan. The overarching goal of this process is selection of treatment strategies and components best suited to meet an individual client's needs before forging ahead with therapy. The following types of information should be considered when developing a treatment plan: idiosyncratic clinical features, interpersonal problems and social support, medical problems and conditions, and the nature of any associated disability, impairment, and quality of life interference.

### *Idiosyncratic Symptom, Cognitive, and Behavioral Features*

Much of the information collected during intake and diagnostic assessment interviews can inform an individual treatment plan. While obtaining a valid DSM-IV diagnosis is indeed one purpose of diagnostic assessment, well-conducted clinical interviews also yield useful idiographic details. As discussed above, the ADIS-IV semi-structured interviews are preferable not only because of their demonstrated diagnostic reliability, but because they contain questions that aid in treatment planning. For example, questions about prominent worry topics ("What kinds of things do you worry about?"), questions about feared outcomes ("Specifically, what types of things do you worry might happen regarding…"), and clinician severity ratings of each somatic symptom help identify an individual's idiosyncratic cognitive and affective features. Client responses to the questionnaire measures reviewed in the previous section may also reveal specific worry topics, meta-cognitive beliefs, and thought control strategies to target in treatment.

Finally, clinicians should assess for any avoidance behavior and worry-related behaviors. Often worry topics will suggest certain avoidance behavior. For example, excessive worry about work might lead to procrastination or avoidance of particular work responsibilities. Worry about the physical safety of loved ones may result in avoidance of watching, reading, or listening to the news. Questions such as "What sorts of things do you do in response to your worries?" or "How do you cope with your anxiety when you're worried?" can reveal any habitual behavior that may reduce discomfort in the short-term but maintain excessive worry in the long term. Common worry-related behaviors include making detailed "to-do" lists, calling others repeatedly to check their safety, reassurance seeking, and checking work repeatedly for accuracy. Some worry-related behaviors are specific to the worry topic, such as an individual routinely leaving home for appointments 30 min early to ensure never being late.

Once an individual's specific symptoms, cognitions, and behavior are identified, these problems can be targeted directly in treatment. For example, clients complaining of muscle tension, aches, and/or soreness can learn to relax their muscles systematically with progressive relaxation techniques. Clients complaining of significant sleep disturbance would likely benefit from adopting a sleep hygiene regimen and practicing cognitive therapy techniques before bedtime. Clients with attention and concentration difficulties may benefit from a number of relaxation strategies that require present-moment focus of attention. Clients prone to overestimating the likelihood of feared events are expected to benefit from cognitive therapy techniques that examine the likelihood of feared events. Likewise, clients who tend to catastrophize the meaning of undesirable outcomes might benefit from decatastrophizing strategies. Meta-cognition, such as beliefs that the person must worry to ward off unwanted events, can be challenged by conducting behavioral experiments. Finally, exposure and response prevention behavior therapy techniques target specific avoidance and worry-related behaviors.

## Interpersonal Problems and Social Support

In addition to client-specific cognitive and behavioral intrapersonal factors, interpersonal and social factors should also be considered. Consistent with growing evidence that GAD individuals report significant interpersonal problems (Borkovec et al. 2002;

Shoenberger & Hazlett-Stevens in press), assessment of the client's interpersonal style of behavior also may be useful. Many clinicians assess interpersonal behavior by taking a detailed psychosocial history during the initial clinical interview and carefully observing clients' social interactions with the therapist. Self-report measures provide another assessment modality. The Inventory of Interpersonal Problems Circumplex Scales (IIP-C; Alden, Wiggins, & Pincus 1990) is a 64-item questionnaire that can detect specific interpersonal styles associated with GAD, such as overly nurturant and intrusive, socially avoidant or nonassertive, and cold or vindictive (Pincus & Borkovec 1994). The IIP-C can help clinicians identify specific interpersonal behavior patterns hindering the formation of supportive relationships and/or the development of intimacy in current relationships. Results from such an assessment might also shed light on the interpersonal dynamics of the therapeutic relationship.

Client descriptions of important personal relationships also can reveal the nature and extent of available social support networks. Social support can be an essential resource as the client undergoes the difficult process of psychotherapy. Furthermore, significant others' reactions to clients' symptoms as well as to changes made during the therapy process can impact treatment outcome dramatically for better or for worse. For this reason, many cognitive-behavioral therapists will involve significant others in treatment to some degree. Finally, assessment of emotional expression and emotion regulation abilities might also inform case conceptualization and treatment planning. As discussed in Chap. 1, emotional regulation deficits might underlie much of the interpersonal distress and negative affect associated with GAD symptoms (Mennin et al. 2004, 2005). Clinicians can choose from a battery of emotion regulation related self-report measures to assess difficulties identifying, describing, and managing emotions. The Difficulties in Emotion Regulation Scale (DERS; Gratz & Roemer 2004) is a promising new measure developed for this purpose. Similar available measures are presented and discussed by Turk and colleagues (2005). Clients exhibiting significant interpersonal and emotion regulation difficulties may benefit from adjunct therapy approaches that target these problems directly.

## Medical Problems and Conditions

Questions about medical history and current medical conditions are included in most diagnostic assessment procedures. Clinicians must rule out general medical conditions as an explanation for GAD symptoms before making the diagnosis. When medical conditions are present but cannot fully account for GAD symptoms, treatment goals might include improved management of chronic medical conditions as well as management of worry and anxiety in response to medical symptoms and concerns. Ideally, the mental health clinician would obtain a signed release from the client and consult with the client's treating physician when medical conditions are present. Consultation with the client's physician can clarify the degree to which certain medical condition(s) may contribute to GAD symptoms and can also help identify any health-related behavior change indicated for that medical condition. In some instances, self-report measures of worry about specific medical conditions may be available. Examples include the Cambridge Worry Scale developed for use with pregnant women (CWS; Green, Kafetsios, Statham, & Snowdon 2003) and the Cancer Worries Inventory developed for use with cancer patients (CWI; D'Errico, Galassi, Schanberg, & Ware 1999). When prominent medical conditions are present, the treatment plan might include cognitive and behavioral strategies that target anxiety, worry, and maladaptive coping responses specific to those medical conditions. Relaxation or other coping strategies for management of physical symptoms and/or behavioral techniques to increase medical treatment adherence might also be warranted.

## *Disability, Impairment, and Quality of Life Interference*

Finally, information regarding the impact of GAD symptoms should be considered. Ways in which anxiety and worry compromise clients' quality of life as well as their social and occupational functioning should be discussed during the clinical interview process. Clients exhibiting difficulty identifying these factors in the interview might complete self-report measures such as the Liebowitz Self-Rated Disability Scale (Schneier, Heckelman, Garfinkel, Campeas et al. 1994), the Sheehan Disability Scale (Sheehan 1983), or the Quality of Life Inventory (QOL; Frisch 1994). See Turk et al. (2004) and Mendlowicz and Stein (2000) for further information about these and similar measures. In some cases, the impairment and interference associated with GAD symptoms might be subtle and somewhat difficult to recognize. For example, the client may be able to work, care for children, and fulfill other major role obligations yet struggle with time management and problem-solving difficulties. Indeed, GAD individuals reported poor problem orientation and little confidence in their problem-solving abilities despite adequate knowledge of problem-solving skills (e.g., Ladouceur, Dugas, Freeston, Rhéaume, et al. 1999). Thus, GAD clients often become so overwhelmed with negative affect that effective problem-solving and time management strategies are not implemented. These various forms of impairment can be incorporated into the treatment plan with specific goals such as returning to work, improved problem solving, or increased frequency of enjoyable activity.

## *Treatment Plan Construction*

Mental health professionals are under increasing pressure to formulate treatment plans with clear objectives and measurable outcomes. Ideally, clients and therapists collaborate during the treatment planning process, with the therapist helping the client identify realistic treatment goals that can be achieved within a certain time frame. After a comprehensive assessment, the therapist and client review prominent factors to target in treatment and generate a problem list. The therapist also describes intervention strategies he or she plans to implement to address each goal, allowing for client informed consent to treatment.

Treatment goals often include reductions in specific symptoms. Reduction in the frequency and intensity of worry is a common example among GAD clients.

However, more detailed changes believed to lead to this clinical outcome also could be articulated. For example, a client reporting strongly-held beliefs that he or she must worry to prevent bad things from happening might benefit from a stated treatment goal of learning to test and challenge positive worry beliefs. Specific cognitive therapy techniques to reduce likelihood overestimation of negative outcomes and catastrophizing, if applicable, should be described. Furthermore, reduction in other somatic anxiety symptoms, such as sleep disturbance, and comorbid symptoms, such as depression, should be included. The specific treatment strategies selected to address each also should be identified and described to the client. Clients expressing severely depressed mood, hopelessness, or suicidal ideation typically need immediate crisis intervention first. Only after stabilization would the therapist proceed to other symptom reduction treatment goals.

In addition to symptom reduction, treatment goals should encompass specific desired behavioral changes identified during the initial assessment process. Examples include reduction or elimination of specific worry maintaining behaviors, such as reassurance seeking, and reductions in behaviors that distract clients from engaging in productive activity and prevent effective time management, such as watching television. Specific interpersonal behaviors, such as increased assertiveness or decreased critical remarks, also should be considered. Other behavioral goals might reflect impaired functioning and quality of life, such as returning to work or school and increased participation in pleasurable leisure activities. Once treatment goals targeting the client's main problem areas have been generated, the therapist and client prioritize each and decide how to proceed with treatment. Therapists should begin treatment only after the client demonstrates a clear understanding of the treatment plan and proposed treatment strategies and has willfully consented to participate.

## Chapter Summary

Diagnostic assessment is a crucial first step when conducting a comprehensive clinical evaluation, largely because the available empirically-supported treatments were developed and tested with individuals meeting GAD diagnostic criteria. Obtaining a reliable GAD diagnosis is only the first step, however. Comprehensive assessment also requires exploration of underlying constructs, such a meta-cognitive beliefs and intolerance of uncertainty. A few of these assessment instruments have been examined among older adults, and two additional self-report worry measures were developed specifically for this population. The diagnostic assessment instruments and measures of worry and worry-related constructs reviewed in this chapter are listed in Table 3.1.

Further information regarding a client's interpersonal functioning, avoidance and other worry-related behavior, and comorbid psychological and medical conditions is needed to create a complete treatment plan that addresses a wide range of concerns. Comprehensive assessments allow for personalized treatment plans tailored to meet the specific needs of each client. A recommended timeline for implementation of the CBT treatment procedures described in this book is provided in Table 3.2.

**Table 3.1** GAD Assessment Measures

| Diagnostic assessment instruments | Worry and related measures |
|---|---|
| **Clinician-administered semi-structured interviews:** | **Self-report measure of worry severity:** |
| *Anxiety Disorders Interview Schedule for DSM-IV (ADIS-IV)* DiNardo, Brown, and Barlow 1994 | *Penn State Worry Questionnaire (PSWQ)* Meyer, Miller, Metzger, and Borkovec 1990 |
| *Structured Clinical Interview for DSM-IV (SCID-I/P)* First et al. 2001 | **Self-report measure of worry content:** *Worry Domains Questionnaire (WDQ)* Tallis, Eysenck, and Mathews 1992 |
| *Schedule for Affective Disorders and Schizophrenia (SADS-LA-IV)* Fyer, Endicott, Mannuza, and Klein 1995 | **Self-report measures of meta-worry:** *Anxious Thoughts Inventory (AnTI)* Wells 1994 *Meta-worry Questionnaire (MWQ)* Wells 2005 |
| **Clinician-administered fully structured interviews:** | **Self-report measures of worry beliefs:** |
| *Diagnostic Interview Schedule, Version IV (DIS-IV)* Robins, Cottler, Bucholz, and Compton 1995 | *Reasons To Worry Questionnaire* Borkovec and Roemer 1995 *Why Worry Scale (WW)* and *Why Worry-II Scale* Freeston, Rhéaume, Letarte, et al. 1994 |
| *Composite International Diagnostic Interview version 2.1 (CIDI)* World Health Organization 1997 | *Consequences of Worry Scale (COWS)* Davey, Tallis, and Capuzzo 1996 |
| **Clinician-administered brief diagnostic interviews:** | **Structured interview measure of worry beliefs:** *Structured Interview on Beliefs About Worry (SIBAW)* Francis and Dugas 2004 |
| *Mini International Neuropsychiatric Interview for DSM-IV (MINI)* Sheehan and Lecrubier 2002 | **Self-report measures of meta-cognitive constructs:** *Meta-Cognitions Questionnaire (MCQ)* Cartwright-Hatton and Wells 1997 |
| *Primary Care Evaluation of Mental Disorders (PRIME-MD)* with *Patient Health Questionnaire* Spitzer, Williams, Kroenke, Linzer, et al. 1994 | *Thought-Action Fusion scale (TAF)* Shafran, Thordarson, and Rachman 1996 *Thought Control Questionnaire (TCQ)* Wells and Davies 1994; Wells 2000 |
| **Diagnostic screening questionnaires:** | *Cognitive Avoidance Questionnaire (CAQ)* Sexton and Dugas 2008 |
| *Psychiatric Diagnostic Screening Questionnaire (PDSQ)* Zimmerman and Mattia 2001a | **Self-report measure of intolerance of uncertainty:** *Intolerance of Uncertainty Scale (IUS)* Freeston, Rhéaume, Letarte, et al. 1994 |
| *Generalized Anxiety Disorder Questionnaire-IV (GAD-Q-IV)* Newman, Zuellig, Kachin, Constantino, et al. 2002 | **Worry measures for older adults:** *Worry Scale for Older Adults (WSOA-R)* Hunt, Wisocki, and Yanko 2003 |
| **Brief clinical interview for older adults:** *Short Anxiety Screening Test (SAST)* Sinoff, Ore, Zlotogorsky, and Tamir 1999 | *Worry Questionnaire for Nursing Home Residents (WQNHR)* Hertzsprung, Konnert, and Brinker 2004 |

**Table 3.2** Suggested Timeline for CBT Procedures

**Session 1:**

Psychoeducation
• GAD information
• Causes of GAD
• Cognitive-behavioral model of GAD
• Definitions of fear, anxiety, and worry
• CBT treatment rationale
• Role of the client in the therapy process
Anxiety self-monitoring rationale
Homework:
Self-monitoring with Anxiety Diary Form

**Session 2:**

Review self-monitoring
Continue or review psychoeducation
Diaphragmatic breathing (DB) rationale
DB session procedures
Initial cognitive therapy procedures
• Cognitive therapy rationale
• Identify specific anxious thoughts
• Thought tracking and worry postponement
Homework:
Self-monitoring with Anxiety Diary Form
Twice daily DB home practice
Thought Tracking Form Step 1

**Session 3:**

Review self-monitoring
Review diaphragmatic breathing home practice
Review Thought Tracking Form Step 1
Progressive relaxation training (PRT) rationale
Initial PRT session procedures
Homework:
Self-monitoring with Anxiety Diary Form
Thought Tracking Form Step 1
Daily formal relaxation home practice
• PRT 16 muscle group practice
• DB practice

**Session 4:**

Review self-monitoring
Review PRT and DB home practice
Review Thought Tracking Form Step 1
Cognitive techniques to challenge anxious
    thoughts
• Generate alternative interpretations or predictions
• Examine likelihood and evidence
• Decatastrophizing
Homework:
Self-monitoring with Anxiety Diary Form
Thought Tracking Form Steps 1–4
(Steps 2–4 conducted during worry period)
Daily formal relaxation home practice
• PRT 16 muscle group practice
• DB practice

**Session 5:**

Review self-monitoring
Review PRT and DB home practice
Review Thought Tracking Form Steps 1–4
Identify worry safety behavior
Identify passive avoidance behavior
Imagery relaxation training rationale
Imagery relaxation training session
    procedures
Homework:
Self-monitoring with Anxiety Diary Form
Thought Tracking Form Steps 1–4
Daily formal relaxation home practice
• PRT 16 muscle group practice
• DB practice
• Imagery relaxation practice
Response prevention for first worry safety
    behavior
First exposure assignment for passive
    avoidance

**Session 6:**

Review self-monitoring
Review relaxation home practice
Review Thought Tracking Form Steps 1–4
Review behavior therapy assignments
Identify and examine core beliefs
Seven muscle group PRT in-session practice
Homework:
Self-monitoring with Anxiety Diary Form
Thought Tracking Form Steps 1–5
Daily formal relaxation home practice
• PRT 7 muscle group practice
• DB practice
• Imagery relaxation practice
Next response prevention assignment
Next exposure assignment

**Session 7:**

Review self-monitoring
Review relaxation home practice
Review Thought Tracking Form Steps 1–5
Review behavior therapy assignments
Continue to identify and examine
    core beliefs
Identify and examine meta-cognitive worry
    beliefs
Introduce imagery exposure and coping
    rehearsal
• Conduct first imagery exposure scene
Homework:
Self-monitoring with Anxiety Diary Form
Thought Tracking Form Steps 1–5
Daily formal relaxation home practice

(continued)

**Table 3.2** (continued)

- PRT 7 muscle group practice
- DB practice
- Imagery relaxation and imagery exposure practice
Next response prevention assignment
Next exposure assignment

**Session 8:**
Review self-monitoring
Review relaxation and imagery exposure practice
Review Thought Tracking Form Steps 1–5
Review behavior therapy assignments
Continue to examine core beliefs
Continue to examine meta-cognitive worry beliefs
Continue imagery exposure and coping rehearsal
- Conduct next imagery exposure scene
Homework:
Self-monitoring with Anxiety Diary Form
Thought Tracking Form Steps 1–5
Daily formal relaxation home practice
- PRT 7 muscle group practice
- DB practice
- Imagery relaxation and imagery exposure practice
Next response prevention assignment
Next exposure assignment

**Session 9:**
Review self-monitoring
Review relaxation and imagery exposure practice
Review Thought Tracking Form Steps 1–5
Review behavior therapy assignments
Continue to examine core beliefs
Continue to examine meta-cognitive worry beliefs
Establish new perspectives
- Develop new perspectives
- Construct preventive beliefs
- Develop coping self-statements
Four muscle group PRT in-session practice
Continue imagery exposure and coping rehearsal
- Conduct next imagery exposure scene
Homework:
Self-monitoring with Anxiety Diary Form
Thought Tracking Form Steps 1–6
Daily formal relaxation home practice
- PRT 4 muscle group practice
- DB practice

- Imagery relaxation and imagery exposure practice
Next response prevention and exposure assignments

**Session 10:**
Review self-monitoring
Review relaxation and imagery exposure practice
Review Thought Tracking Form Steps 1–6
Review behavior therapy assignments
Continue to examine core beliefs
Continue to examine meta-cognitive worry beliefs
Lifestyle behavior change
- Identify neglected activities
Continue imagery exposure and coping rehearsal
- Conduct next imagery exposure scene
Homework:
Self-monitoring with Anxiety Diary Form
Thought Tracking Form Steps 1–6
Daily formal relaxation home practice
- PRT 4 muscle group practice
- DB practice
- Imagery relaxation and imagery exposure practice
Any remaining behavior therapy assignments
Engage in desired activity

**Session 11:**
Review self-monitoring
Review relaxation and imagery exposure practice
Review Thought Tracking Form Steps 1–6
Review behavior therapy assignments
Review desired activity engagement
Continue to examine core beliefs
Continue to examine meta-cognitive worry beliefs
PRT relaxation recall procedures
Continue imagery exposure and coping rehearsal
- Conduct next imagery exposure scene
Homework:
Self-monitoring with Anxiety Diary Form
Thought Tracking Form Steps 1–6
Daily formal relaxation home practice
- PRT relaxation recall practice
- DB practice
- Imagery relaxation and imagery exposure practice
Any remaining behavior therapy assignments
Engage in desired activity

(continued)

**Table 3.2** (continued)

**Session 12:**

Review self-monitoring

Review relaxation and imagery exposure practice

Review Thought Tracking Form Steps 1–6

Review behavior therapy assignments

Review desired activity engagement

Continue to examine core beliefs

Continue to examine meta-cognitive worry beliefs

PRT relaxation recall by counting procedures

Continue imagery exposure and coping rehearsal

• Conduct next imagery exposure scene

Homework:

Self-monitoring with Anxiety Diary Form

Thought Tracking Form Steps 1–6

Daily formal relaxation home practice

• PRT relaxation recall by counting practice

• DB practice

• Imagery relaxation and imagery exposure practice

Any remaining behavior therapy assignments

Engage in desired activity

**Session 13:**

Review self-monitoring

Review relaxation and imagery exposure practice

Review Thought Tracking Form Steps 1–6

Review behavior therapy assignments

Review desired activity engagement

Continue to examine core beliefs

Continue to examine meta-cognitive worry beliefs

Applied relaxation procedures

• Relaxation coping responses

• Relaxation reminder cues

• Daily brief relaxation practice

Continue imagery exposure and coping rehearsal

• Conduct next imagery exposure scene

Homework:

Self-monitoring with Anxiety Diary Form

Thought Tracking Form Steps 1–6

Daily formal relaxation home practice

• PRT relaxation recall by counting practice

• DB practice

• Imagery relaxation and imagery exposure practice

Applied relaxation practice

Any remaining behavior therapy assignments

Engage in desired activity

**Session 14:**

Review previous home assignments

Continue previous therapy components as needed

Introduce relapse prevention

• Review client progress

• Review essential psychoeducation information

Homework:

Self-monitoring with Anxiety Diary Form

Thought Tracking Form Steps 1–6

Daily formal relaxation home practice

• PRT relaxation recall by counting practice

• DB practice

• Imagery relaxation and imagery exposure practice

Applied relaxation practice

Any remaining behavior therapy assignments

Engage in desired activity

**Session 15:**

Review previous home assignments

Continue previous therapy components as needed

Continue relapse prevention planning

• Continued practice plan for therapy skills

• Construct written relapse prevention plan

Homework:

Applied relaxation practice

Engage in desired activity

Any remaining therapy assignments

**Session 16:**

Review previous home assignments

Continue previous therapy components as needed

Finalize relapse prevention planning

• Review written relapse prevention plan

Homework:

Application of relapse prevention plan

# Chapter 4
# Psychoeducation and Anxiety Monitoring

Cognitive-behavioral therapy (CBT) for GAD is based on the premise that clients have learned maladaptive patterns of perceiving and responding to their environments and therefore lack effective coping strategies. From this perspective, GAD clients are suffering from excessive worry and anxiety because they are prone to perceive threat and respond with avoidance and inaction rather than constructive behavior. After years of identifying potential threats and responding with worry, anxiety, and avoidance, these clients have developed habitual and automatic response patterns. Anxious thoughts, sensations, and behavior are rehearsed so often that these sequences eventually occur completely out of awareness.

The various CBT treatment components aim to interrupt this vicious cycle at different points. Cognitive restructuring strategies directly target inflated perceptions of threat and beliefs that the client would be unable to cope with feared situations or outcomes. Progressive relaxation and deep breathing techniques teach new physical responses to somatic cues such as muscle tension and shallow breathing. Relaxation strategies also can be incorporated into a client's daily routine to decrease baseline anxiety and tension levels, reducing the chances that anxious response cycles will develop in the first place. Finally, behavior therapy techniques such as response prevention and exposure target specific safety and avoidance behaviors. Worry-related safety behaviors, such as reassurance seeking, and passive avoidance of feared situations further increase perceptions of threat. Crucially, such behavior also precludes corrective learning experiences; clients deprive themselves of opportunities to experience first-hand what would have happened and how they would have coped had they stayed in the feared situation without engaging in safety behaviors.

Based on this cognitive-behavioral model, the CBT treatment approach requires that clients first understand the underlying theoretical model and identify their own personal response patterns. Similar to cognitive-behavioral therapies for other clinical problems, CBT for GAD begins with a psychoeducation component. In addition to background information about GAD diagnosis and symptoms, clients are presented with a cognitive-behavioral model to provide a framework for understanding their symptoms and anxious experience. Differences between adaptive and excessive anxiety are discussed to address any misguided expectations that therapy will simply rid clients of anxiety altogether. Psychoeducation is considered an essential

H. Hazlett-Stevens, *Psychological Approaches to Generalized Anxiety Disorder*,
doi: 10.1007/978-0-387-76870-0, © Springer Science + Business Media, LLC 2008

initial treatment component for several reasons. First, clients' understanding of the treatment rationale generates necessary motivation to invest their time and effort in treatment sessions and completing homework assignments. Second, an appreciation for how treatment procedures are believed to lead to desirable therapy outcomes fosters positive client expectancies and instills hope. Finally, early psychoeducation discussions provide therapists the opportunity to establish rapport and build a strong collaborative therapeutic alliance from the beginning.

Frequent client self-monitoring of anxiety levels, anxiety cues and triggers, and relevant thoughts, sensations, and behavior is also recommended at the outset of treatment. Most cognitive-behavioral therapists view regular self-monitoring as the foundation for all future interventions. Anxiety is conceptualized as the result of automatic and habitual patterns of responding. Therefore, clients first must become aware of their own idiosyncratic response patterns. Otherwise, interruption of problematic anxiety cycles by intervening with a new coping response is not possible. In addition to increased self-awareness, self-monitoring exercises help clients learn to distance themselves from their anxious experience. Clients view their anxious thoughts, sensations, and behavior more objectively, allowing for a sense of choice over subsequent reactions. Self-monitoring also provides the therapist with in-the-moment data to monitor the client's progress each week. Clinical information obtained this way is often more accurate and reliable than a retrospective account of the past week reported at the beginning of a session. Many times a client will begin the session describing a horrible week filled with anxiety and worry, only to realize that this global impression was based on just one or two particularly difficult days. In these cases, self-monitoring data allow clients to discover their own retrospective memory biases and tendencies to over-generalize negative experiences.

Finally, self-monitoring data help the therapist and client identify certain times of day or days of the week when the client is most vulnerable to episodes of excessive worry and anxiety. Such discoveries can lead to future intervention around problematic situations when coping strategies might be most useful. For example, consider the case of a client who consistently recorded increases in anxiety coming home from work each day. Exploration of anxious thoughts during her drive home revealed high levels of anticipatory anxiety over caring for her young children while preparing dinner in time for the rest of her family. Cognitive and problem-solving strategies around this issue proved helpful. In addition, the client experimented with the timing of her relaxation practice. She soon discovered that 5 min of progressive relaxation and deep breathing alone in her bedroom before paying the childcare worker significantly reduced her anxiety levels for the rest of the evening.

Psychoeducation and self-monitoring provide the foundation for all other active CBT components. Therefore, this information is presented at the beginning of treatment, typically during the first one or two sessions. These critical treatment elements are also incorporated throughout the later treatment sessions. Therapists remind clients of important cognitive-behavioral principles and review relevant psychoeducation information as appropriate throughout treatment. Likewise, continued self-monitoring is recommended over the entire course of treatment to ensure effective implementation of coping strategies and assessment of therapy progress. This chapter outlines the major points to convey to clients during initial CBT sessions and contains suggestions for presenting this information effectively.

## Psychoeducation

Typically, the first treatment session following assessment and client consent to treatment begins with a discussion of the GAD diagnosis. Various factors that may have led to the development of GAD symptoms are reviewed, and a cognitive-behavioral model of GAD is presented. Clients are encouraged to identify how their own anxious experience fits within this model, and important differences between adaptive and excessive anxiety and worry are clarified. Finally, the therapist explains the treatment rationale, how specific CBT procedures will be implemented, and what is required of the client for therapy to be effective.

### *GAD Information*

Therapists often initiate discussion of GAD diagnosis by asking clients if they have ever heard the term "generalized anxiety disorder" and, if so, what they've learned about GAD so far. Therapists then respond by correcting any misconceptions and highlighting essential diagnostic features. Therapists explain that while everyone experiences anxiety and worry to some degree on occasion, GAD may be diagnosed when worry is excessive, chronic, and difficult to control. This worry covers a variety of topics rather than focusing on only one area of a person's life. In addition, chronic physical symptoms such as restlessness, fatigue, sleep problems, trouble concentrating, irritability, and muscle tension result. The worry and associated anxiety symptoms have grown to the point that they are causing significant distress and/or interfering with the person's life. Often a lack of confidence and interpersonal problems accompany the diagnostic symptoms. When covering this information in session, therapists emphasize particular symptoms and clinical features most salient for that individual client. Therapists also encourage each client to reflect on how the information presented seems consistent as well as inconsistent with the client's own experience.

Therapists then present background facts and statistics about GAD. Epidemiological research results are provided, such as prevalence rates, gender ratio, typical course and onset, and common comorbid psychological and medical conditions. This information is best presented in a conversational, lay-language format. For example, rather than stating that "the lifetime prevalence of GAD is estimated at 5–6%," the therapist might mention that "over 5% of Americans suffer from GAD during their lifetime. This means that about four million adults here in the U.S. alone will struggle with the same sort of symptoms you are experiencing." Again, therapists should encourage clients to reflect upon how the epidemiological information fits or contrasts with their own experience. Has the client felt like a "worrier" all of his/her life or did the worry and anxiety develop during a stressful time in young adulthood? Does the client also struggle with social anxiety, depression, and/or common comorbid medical conditions such as irritable bowel syndrome (IBS)? The more the therapist can personalize this discussion to help the client become aware of his or her own clinical situation, the more meaningful this epidemiological information will seem to the client.

GAD diagnosis and epidemiology are usually discussed in treatment to help clients appreciate that they "are not alone." When asked how they feel during these discussions, clients often express comfort in learning about others like them. Reports of feeling less isolated are also common. This initial clinical intervention therefore serves to address attributions that clients are weak, strange, or "crazy" because they suffer from GAD. Sharing this information often instills hope; clients realize that their therapist already has a working understanding of their problems as well as effective therapy methods to help them. Sometimes, however, clients will experience these discussions as invalidating or stigmatizing. Receiving the diagnosis feels like being labeled, and being told one has a "disorder" feels dehumanizing or demoralizing. In these cases discussion of diagnosis leaves the client feeling misunderstood, as if he or she is not a unique human being with real problems. Thus, an important practice during this intervention involves eliciting client reactions during the discussion. If a client does not immediately respond with a sense of relief, further inquiry about how the client felt upon hearing that he or she received a GAD diagnosis should follow. The therapist might facilitate client disclosure of negative responses by suggesting that "sometimes when people hear about their diagnosis, they actually feel worse" and asking if the client noticed any negative reactions. The therapist might also acknowledge that the diagnostic label, while helpful to guide the therapist in treatment planning, only describes the client's symptoms. The client is a multi-faceted human being, the essence of which cannot be captured by a diagnosis or label.

## Causes of GAD

Clients naturally often wonder why they developed GAD in the first place. Therapists may ask their clients to describe their own personal theories of how and why their symptoms came about, underscoring information supported by research while clarifying any misconceptions. For example, some clients may have heard that GAD is "genetic." Therapists would then explain the notion of a nonspecific genetic predisposition. That is, GAD is very different from a genetically-caused disease. Only a general tendency to react to situations with heightened emotions is genetically inherited. People who inherit this tendency are more prone to experience problems with anxiety or depression than people who do not, but many people inherit this tendency and never have a psychological disorder.

Experiences with other people and the environment are equally, if not more, important. Asking clients what childhood and other past experiences might have contributed to their tendency to worry can lead to fruitful discussions about critical learning experiences. Many situations could result in the fundamental beliefs that the world is dangerous and unpredictable and that one is not capable of protecting him or herself from danger and coping with adversity. Physical and/or sexual abuse, other past trauma or extreme stress, loss of a parent or other caregiver during childhood, and social trauma such as being bullied by a peer are clear examples. Not surprisingly, parenting practices and other parental behavior can have a strong impact. Many parents might model anxious behavior for their children, inadvertently sending the message that the world contains many dangers. Messages of danger are also transmitted when parents express their worries to their children directly or have overprotective rules for their children.

Results from a few adult attachment investigations (Cassidy 1995; Schut, Pincus, Castonguay, Bedics et al. 1997; Zuellig, Newman, Kachin, & Constantino 1997) suggested that a child's perceived relationship to his or her primary caregiver might be linked to adult GAD later in life. Retrospective reports of insecure attachment, particularly when a parent was experienced as critical and/or lacking warmth, were quite common among adults with GAD. One particular child-parent relationship was identified among individuals with GAD: a role-reversed enmeshed relationship. In these cases, clients felt as thought they were responsible for taking care of a parent rather than feeling as though their parents were in charge of taking care of them. As clients describe their childhood relationships with parents or other important caregivers, therapists might help clients identify how such early relationships may have led to reliance on worry as a strategy to cope with unpredictable, uncertain, and uncontrollable situations as well as with difficult emotions.

Cognitive-behavioral therapists vary in the degree to which they discuss their clients' past experiences in treatment. However, some attention to this information might prove useful for a number of reasons. First, therapists often strengthen rapport by anticipating clients' curiosity about themselves and engaging in such a discussion. Many clients come to therapy with the desire to understand themselves better in addition to achieve symptom reduction. Second, insight gained from this brief personal exploration may soften any negative judgments clients have about themselves. Clients adopt alternative explanations for their symptoms that contradict previous beliefs that people suffer from GAD because they are weak, personally flawed, or otherwise at fault. Third, genetic and environmental contributions to GAD are the cornerstone of leading cognitive behavioral models. These influences comprise the biological and psychological vulnerabilities presented in the next psychoeducation segment.

## Cognitive-Behavioral Model of GAD

Therapists next present a working model of how various etiological factors combine, ultimately leading to GAD experience. One popular model has been described by Barlow and colleagues (Roemer, Orsillo, & Barlow 2002). First, GAD individuals may have a propensity to react to situations with anxiety, other negative emotions, and heightened physiological arousal. This generalized tendency, sometimes referred to as "negative affectivity" or "neuroticism," may be partially inherited genetically but is not specific to GAD. This tendency is only considered a diathesis, leaving a person vulnerable to emotional disorders involving anxiety or depression if stressful life events later occur. In such cases, the tendency to experience heightened anxious arousal interacts with the stressful event(s), producing intense levels of anxiety. Such neurotic tendencies may also result from a learning history in which unwanted events were perceived as unpredictable and uncontrollable. As biological and psychological vulnerabilities interact with stressful life events, a state of anxious apprehension involving increased tension and hypervigilance to threat result. These individuals soon learn to see threat easily, often interpreting ambiguous or neutral situations as potentially threatening. Fundamental beliefs that the world is a dangerous place and that one is unable to respond to adversity develop. Worry becomes the primary strategy to cope with perceived threats as the individual attempts to gain control over potential threats as well as spiraling tension and anxious arousal. Failed attempts to gain control lead to distorted cognitive processing, which inhibits effective problem-solving and constructive action. Incorporating aspects of the worry theory described below (Borkovec, Alcaine, & Behar 2004), the avoidance of worry-related images is believed to restrict autonomic response, and the worry process is negatively reinforced by the absence of catastrophic outcomes. Full GAD develops when this worry process becomes so chronic that associated somatic symptoms and clinically severe distress and impairment result.

Therapists then might explain essential features of Borkovec and colleagues' (2004) avoidance theory of worry further. This theory elucidates how worry functions as an attempt to cope with future threat and why counterproductive worry habits strengthen over time. Worry is conceptualized as a cognitive attempt to avoid future danger. When future threat is detected and behavioral avoidance of the threat is not possible, only cognitive activity remains as an available method of avoidance. Future threat may be avoided if ways to prevent the threatening event from occurring or ways to reduce its negative impact can be identified in advance. However, many anticipated negative events may be highly unlikely and therefore would not have occurred anyway. In either case, the worry is negatively reinforced much like other forms of avoidance behavior. Indeed, Borkovec, Hazlett-Stevens, and Diaz (1999) found that GAD individuals reported positive outcomes 85% of the time when asked to track the actual outcomes of worry-related future events. Furthermore, when feared outcomes did occur, better-than-expected coping was reported 79% of the time. In addition to perceived avoidance of threatening events or their consequences, worry may suppress physiological activation and dampen intense experience of fear and other negative emotions. Worry generates unwanted anxiety, distress, and associated symptoms. Nevertheless, this cognitive activity persists in the service of circumventing feared outcomes and suppressing more intense emotional experience. Cognitive beliefs that such constant worry and hypervigilance are necessary for survival often result, further perpetuating a vicious cycle of perceived threats and cognitive avoidance attempts.

## *Definitions of Fear, Anxiety, and Worry*

Once clients have gained insight into how their GAD symptoms may have developed, therapists initiate discussion of how GAD experiences differ from the "normal" anxiety and worry all people face. Fear is described as a basic human emotion we all experience when confronted with immediate physical danger. The "fight-or-flight" response is described as a natural physiological response designed to help us escape from life-threatening dangers at a moment's notice. Thus, the physiological arousal we experience when afraid has evolved so that we can run from or fight the threat effectively. For example, the heart pounds and races to deliver oxygen-rich blood to large muscle groups quickly.

Unlike true fear, anxiety is experienced in anticipation of threat. When we look ahead and see a potential threat in the future, our bodies still react to some degree. Subjective feelings of discomfort and unease accompany the physiological sensations, and these experiences are often interpreted as evidence that the threat is coming and likely to occur. Anxious thoughts about perceived threat interact with physical sensations and behavior to perpetuate anxious experience. In short, anxiety is made up of several different components, including thoughts, physical sensations, subjective feelings, and behaviors. Although anxiety seems to come on suddenly or unexpectedly, anxiety is actually a process that develops over time. People do not notice their anxiety building until it reaches a very high level because the sequences of anxious thoughts, sensations, feelings, and behavior have been rehearsed so often they now occur out of awareness. Once the client recognizes anxiety as an automatic spiral of interactions between thoughts, body sensations, feelings, and behavior, the therapist and client identify the client's own idiosyncratic sequences. The therapist might ask the client to describe a recent episode of anxiety then follow up with specific questions about the individual thoughts, sensations, and behavior the client experienced as the anxiety process unfolded.

During this description of anxiety, therapists acknowledge that anxiety also can be adaptive and useful. Discussion of why humans evolved with the capacity to anticipate danger and react with anxiety should also occur. CBT therapists often describe the seminal research findings of Yerkes and Dodson (1908), who first demonstrated that an optimal amount of arousal actually improved task performance. According to the Yerkes-Dodson Law, performance increases as arousal increases up to a certain point. Performance deteriorates only after the optimal point is reached as the arousal becomes excessive. Clients may be able to recall times in which anxiety served to sharpen their thinking, aiding them in a job interview, first date, class presentation, athletic competition, or other performance situation. Anxiety is only considered a problem when it occurs in excess of the situation at hand. In other words, anxiety is excessive when it interferes with performance and functioning. CBT for GAD is based on the premise that clients are experiencing too much anxious arousal in a variety of situations. While the aim of therapy is to help clients reduce and manage excessive anxiety, clients will continue to experience normative levels of anxiety throughout their lifetime. Clients need to understand that anxiety is fundamentally adaptive at normal levels to adjust any unrealistic expectations that therapy will rid them of anxiety altogether.

Worry is defined as a specific type of anxious thinking in which a person anticipates threat, often by asking "what if" something were to happen, and views him or herself as unable to cope. These future threats might involve physical danger, but often entail social threats such as negative judgments or disapproval of other people. As the person continues to worry about possible negative outcomes, the anxiety spiral grows. However, much like fear and anxiety, worry has adaptive origins. The human ability to think ahead into the future and play out possible scenarios beforehand is essential to our survival. Although worry is excessive and difficult to control for some people, most people worry to some degree from time to time. The crucial factor is how easily a person shifts into concrete problem solving about the situation at hand. Worry soon subsides when it motivates a person to act, thereby providing a solution to a specific problem. People with GAD who worry excessively tend to rely on worry to solve unsolvable problems or to try and prevent outcomes that are unlikely to happen in the first place. In these cases, worry generates anxiety instead of constructive action and problem resolution. At this point, the client might be able to identify times in which thinking ahead led to constructive problem solving instead of excessive anxiety. The therapist could then ask the client to describe how such experiences differed from those in which unproductive worry led to intense anxiety.

## *CBT Treatment Rationale*

Therapists next explain how the different CBT strategies will address the respective components of the anxiety spiral. Clients will first learn to monitor their anxiety and its cognitive, physiological, and behavioral components in an objective way. This regular self-monitoring provides opportunities to interrupt automatic anxiety spirals with various coping strategies.

Relaxation strategies are an important first step to interrupt anxiety spirals by letting go of anxious thoughts and sensations. Clients will learn three different relaxation techniques to prevent unnecessary tension and anxiety from building. Progressive relaxation is a systematic procedure that teaches clients to purposefully tense and release individual muscle groups. With practice, clients will become able to notice and relax away even the slightest bit of muscle tension. Diaphragmatic breathing is a deep breathing technique believed to produce many physiological and cognitive effects, all of which make anxiety spirals less likely to develop. This simple technique involves breathing deeply from the abdomen in place of the shallow chest breathing that has become habitual for most people with GAD. Relaxation through mental imagery teaches clients to use their own imaginations to generate states of subjective and physical relaxation. In addition to practicing and developing effective relaxation skills, clients will learn how to incorporate these new skills into their daily routine.

Cognitive restructuring strategies are based on the premise that anxiety is often caused by perceptions of threat and views of oneself as unable to cope. Cognitive strategies teach clients how to identify specific anxious thoughts and treat those thoughts as mere guesses or predictions. Importantly, clients will learn how to view their situation differently and choose their response rather than simply reacting to the anxious thought as though it were fact. With the help of their therapist, clients will also evaluate thoughts and beliefs about their need to worry and learn to recognize the difference between useful problem solving and unproductive worry.

Finally, behavioral strategies will encourage clients to act differently. Anxiety spiral behavior reduces anxiety in the short term, but strengthens anxiety spirals in the long term. These behaviors reinforce perceptions of threat. Furthermore, clients deprive themselves of experiencing first-hand what would have happened and how they would have coped if they resisted their avoidance urges and faced the feared situation without engaging in safety behaviors. Clients therefore will learn how to confront situations they currently avoid, give up safety behaviors that perpetuate worry and perceptions of threat, and engage in leisure activities and self-care behaviors that GAD clients tend to neglect. They also will practice their new coping strategies in difficult situations with an imagery exposure technique called "self-control desensitization." This final technique provides in-session opportunities to confront feared upcoming situations in imagery while practicing newly learned coping responses such as applied relaxation and cognitive restructuring. This imagery practice will increase the likelihood that clients will remember to use their coping strategies when similar situations arise in daily life.

Once clients have a clear understanding of the individual CBT components, treatment effectiveness is briefly discussed. Therapists summarize the research providing empirical support for this approach to treatment. Approximately 20 state-of-the-art research investigations known as randomized control trials already have been conducted (see Chap. 2 for a review of this literature). Results form these studies are quite consistent, showing that CBT often led to significant reductions in anxiety and depression symptoms. These benefits tended to last after therapy ended, as therapy gains were maintained at 1-year follow-up assessments. Clients receiving CBT were more likely to improve than clients who received no treatment, nondirective counseling, and in some studies, individual cognitive or behavioral treatment components instead of the CBT package.

## *Role of the Client in the Therapy Process*

The psychoeducation component of treatment concludes with a discussion of the client's role in treatment. Before proceeding with the remaining intervention components, clients must understand that effective treatment outcomes depend on their commitment to change and active participation in treatment. This commitment involves regular session attendance, effortful participation in homework exercises and coping strategy practice, and a willingness to try different behaviors. Therapists ask clients about any possible impediments to successful treatment outcomes as well as any resources that might facilitate desired change. Significant interpersonal relationships can function in either direction, either by enabling client avoidance behavior or by providing positive encouragement for behavior change. Scheduling and time management difficulties that might prevent completion of homework exercises also might be anticipated and discussed ahead of time. As McCabe and Antony (2005) suggested for treatment of panic disorder, clients ambivalent about their commitment to CBT procedures might benefit from motivational interviewing techniques (Miller & Rollnick 2002). Clients also should be warned that therapy effects are not immediate. Continued effort and patience, especially at first, are needed before treatment gains appear. In addition, therapy gains typically are not linear. Clients might begin to see some benefit followed by brief setbacks or a return of symptoms.

Finally, therapists can suggest a specific way clients might approach treatment: with an open mind and a sense of curiosity about what might happen. Extreme pessimism usually creates a self-fulfilling prophecy. Clients who expect therapy to fail may practice at first but abandon their efforts at the first sign of difficulty. At the other extreme, clients will soon be disappointed if they hold unrealistic beliefs that CBT will suddenly solve all their problems and spare them the occasional distress and anxiety we all face. Alternatively, clients are encouraged to suspend such judgments until they develop coping strategies and see for themselves whether or not CBT is helpful to them. This discussion introduces the "collaborative empiricism" approach crucial for effective cognitive therapy (Beck, Rush, Shaw, & Emery 1979). Rather than jumping to conclusions, assumptions about the future are treated as mere predictions. Such judgments can only be trusted after the events in question have occurred and objective evidence has been collected.

## Style of Presentation

Therapists are faced with a difficult dilemma during the initial psychoeducation therapy sessions. The need to present clients with a large volume of information must be balanced with therapeutic relationship building and rapport. Therapists often feel pressed to get through psychoeducation material quickly so that coping strategies can be taught as early as feasible to reduce client distress. One possible solution is to provide clients with reading material beforehand. Clients are given self-help guides, workbooks, or handouts summarizing essential psychoeducation information during informed consent to treatment. Clients then return to therapy already having read this information, allowing the session to focus on discussion and clarification of material. A number of reading options have been published for this purpose. Two self-help books specifically targeting the chronic worry seen in GAD recently have been released: *Women who worry too much* (Hazlett-Stevens 2005) and *The worry cure* (Leahy 2005a). A client workbook and accompanying therapist guide entitled *Mastery of your anxiety and worry, 2nd edition* were developed by Craske, Barlow, and colleagues (MAW-2; Craske & Barlow 2006a; Zinbarg,

Craske, & Barlow 2006). Finally, a single-page summary client handout appears in Leahy and Holland (2000, pp. 125–126), and a more comprehensive four-page client handout is provided by Rygh and Sanderson (2004, pp. 59–62). Therapists either can provide clients with one of these resources or construct their own handout containing essential psychoeducation information.

Regardless of whether or not clients read psychoeducation information on their own beforehand, therapists should avoid a didactic presentation style whenever possible. A didactic style might be necessary to some degree when presenting to large groups in a workshop format, but attempts should be made to involve group members in discussion as much as possible. Lecturing to individual or small group therapy clients might inadvertently alter the therapeutic dynamic, establishing a hierarchical relationship more so than a collaborative one. Furthermore, clients are more likely to retain psychoeducation material when elicited from them rather than told to them (Zinbarg et al. 2006). Consider the following two hypothetical individual therapy transcripts. Both involve discussion of the cognitive, physiological, and behavioral components of anxiety. However, the therapist presents this information in an interactive and desirable way only in the second example.

Transcript #1 (Didactic presentation style):

Therapist: Now I'd like to talk about the nature of anxiety. Anxiety is an emotion we all experience in anticipation of threat. When we look ahead and see a potential threat in the future, our bodies react in certain ways. Common physical sensations include muscle tension, stomach distress, accelerated heart rate, and many others. Subjective feelings of discomfort are part of anxiety too, such as unease, feeling on edge, or irritability. Do you have any questions?

Client: No, not really.

T: Okay. Anxious thoughts, or what you say to yourself when you're anxious, are important too. Thoughts about perceived threat interact with physical sensations and behavior to perpetuate anxious experience. In other words, anxiety is made up of several different components, including thoughts, physical sensations, subjective feelings, and behaviors. Anxious behavior usually involves some sort of avoidance, like avoiding a particular situation or activity related to your worry and anxiety.

Transcript #2 (Interactive presentation style):

Therapist: Let's talk a bit about what anxiety is. How do you know when you're feeling anxious?

Client: What do you mean? I just feel it.

T: Take right now, for example. How anxious are you feeling? On a scale from 0 to 100, where 0 is completely relaxed with no anxiety at all, and 100 is absolutely terrified, how would you rate how you're feeling at the moment?

C: Not too bad...I guess about 50.

T: Okay, a 50. What experiences did you tune into to come up with that rating? In other words, what thoughts, bodily sensations, or feelings did you notice?

C: Well…my shoulders are kind of scrunched up and tense. And now that I'm thinking about it, I realize I'm clenching my jaw.

T: Good, so you notice anxiety in your body and your muscles. What else do you notice?

C: Um…my stomach is a little queasy. I feel a little on edge.

T: So anxiety is really made up of a combination of experiences: different physical sensations in your body as well as subjective feelings like being on edge. Anxiety is an emotion everyone feels when they think that something threatening or problematic might be coming. Did you notice any anxious thoughts going through your mind? What were you saying to yourself just before you rated your anxiety at 50?

C: What if I'm not smart enough to do this. I guess I was wondering if I'll be able to learn all that you're trying to teach me and not feeling too confident about it.

T: Sounds like some anxious thoughts about the future and specifically about you not having the ability to benefit from treatment. As you'll see down the road, this therapy working has much more to do with the effort and dedication you put in than book smarts. We'll be sure to talk about that issue some more before we end today. But notice how those thoughts contributed to your anxiety. Thoughts about the future can play a huge role in how anxious you feel. What's important to realize is that anxiety is made up of several components: thoughts, bodily sensations, feelings, and even behavior. How about anxious behavior? What do you tend to do when you're anxious?

C: Well, I don't tend to do much. When I get very anxious and worried, I'll usually just sit on the couch watching TV and not really do anything about it.

T: So you'll respond by not taking much action, or avoiding the situation.

C: Exactly.

## Anxiety Monitoring

Frequent client monitoring of anxiety levels, internal and external triggers, and the specific thoughts, subjective feelings, physical sensations, and behavior that comprise anxiety spirals should begin as early as feasible in treatment. Therapists first present a rationale for self-monitoring, followed by a description of self-monitoring homework procedures and specific instructions for recording this information between sessions. In addition, therapists model frequent monitoring during therapy sessions with repeated requests for in-the-moment client anxiety ratings.

### *Self-Monitoring Rationale*

Therapists first explain the value of self-monitoring to foster clients' willingness and compliance. This rationale begins with a review of the anxiety spiral, in which anxiety episodes are described as sequences of events that take place much like a chain reaction. Each reaction to the previous reaction has been rehearsed so frequently, these anxiety spirals have become automatic and often occur out of awareness. Below is a hypothetical therapy transcript presenting this initial information:

Therapist: Throughout this treatment it is very important that you learn to monitor your level of anxiety frequently. The goal is for you to become more and more aware of even the smallest shifts in your anxiety level over time. How do you think self-monitoring might be useful to you?

Client: Well, this might help me become more aware of what's going on inside...usually I don't even understand why I'm so anxious.

T: Exactly! Anxiety often seems to come on suddenly or unexpectedly...we often don't notice it building until it reaches a very high level. But with careful monitoring you'll see that anxiety is actually a *process*. In other words, anxiety is made up of a series of thoughts, sensations, feelings, and behaviors, each happening in reaction to the previous one. Think back over your own anxiety episodes this past week. Can you think of an example?

C: Yes, last Tuesday at work I felt especially anxious all morning. By the time my lunch hour came around I was a mess.

T: Okay...let's start at the beginning. When did you first notice you were feeling anxious?

C: Well, I had a sense of dread before I even got to my desk as I was walking into work from the parking lot.

T: What might have triggered your anxiety? Were you thinking about anything in particular?

C: Oh yeah, I was worrying about the 10:00 monthly staff meeting.

T: So this feeling of dread was a reaction to anxious thoughts. What exactly were you saying to yourself about the meeting?

C: What if I get put on the spot? The branch supervisor might ask me to report on our budget.

T: And what about that worried you? What were you concerned might happen?

C: That I'd fumble my words or forget to mention something important. Then my boss would think I didn't prepare for the meeting.

T: It sounds like that particular anxiety spiral began with an anxious thought about your meeting. How were you feeling the moment before you remembered that you had the meeting that morning?

C: Fine, at least no different from usual.

T: So this episode was triggered by a thought...you remembered the meeting, which triggered anxious thoughts about not performing well in the meeting and looking unprepared in front of your boss. These thoughts then led to that subjective feeling of dread. What happened next?

[As the therapist and client explored this situation, the client identified a series of physical sensations, catastrophic thoughts both before and after the meeting, and worry-related behavior of repeatedly seeking reassurance from a trusted co-worker. By noon, the client's anxiety level had increased to 70 and she felt like her stomach was in knots.]

T: Notice how your anxiety involved a spiral of interactions between your thoughts, body sensations, feelings, and behavior. As you interacted with the world around you over the course of the morning, your anxiety steadily increased up to its peak of 70. But at the time your anxiety felt like one big mass of discomfort and you weren't really aware of all these moment-to-moment reactions. That's because these sequences of reactions become very automatic, like habits you've developed from the past. Each time an anxiety spiral experience like this happens, it gets stored in your memory and this automatic habit gets stronger.

[The therapist and client then explored the client's typical sequence of anxious thoughts, sensations, subjective feelings, and behavior characterizing her anxiety spirals. This led to a fruitful discussion of how the client usually responded to early cues of anxiety and how such automatic reactions often encouraged development of anxiety spirals.]

Therapists conclude the self-monitoring rationale with an explanation of its many purposes. Below are several reasons to self-monitor therapists raise with their clients:

1. Frequent monitoring teaches clients to view their anxious thoughts, subjective feelings, sensations, and behavior more objectively, allowing for a sense of choice over subsequent reactions. Clients become objective observers of their responses and behavior to develop a greater understanding of anxious experience.
2. With frequent monitoring, clients learn to detect subtle increases in anxiety. When clients notice small shifts in anxiety or distress, they enable themselves to catch anxiety spirals developing early. Coping strategies can then be deployed as early as possible, preventing further development of the anxiety spiral. In addition, the earlier in the anxiety process a coping strategy is used, the easier the strategy will be to implement. Repeated practice builds new coping response habits in place of old anxiety spiral habits.
3. Self-monitoring also helps clients identify common anxiety spiral triggers. Both internal and external events can trigger anxiety outside of awareness. As clients become more and more skilled at identifying triggers, their anxiety spirals can be prevented with alternative responses to these cues or events.
4. Self-monitoring records provide therapists information about client experiences outside of therapy sessions. This information helps therapists monitor client progress over the course of treatment. In addition, self-monitoring data recorded in-the-moment tends to be more objective and accurate than retrospective reports which are subject to mood-dependent recall (Zinbarg et al. 2006).
5. Finally, self-monitoring records help therapists and clients identify patterns of anxiety levels over time. Vulnerable periods of time, such as certain times of day

or certain days of the week, are then targeted for intervention. Clients can make a special effort to implement coping strategies during these vulnerable times when coping responses are expected to be most useful.

## Within-Session Modeling of Frequent Monitoring

In addition to the self-monitoring homework described below, therapists model frequent monitoring during therapy sessions. Near the beginning of each therapy session, therapists ask clients to rate their current anxiety level. Therapists can use the 0–100 scale described above or any other rating scale that corresponds to the self-monitoring forms selected for homework. Each time a client reports an anxiety rating, the therapist asks follow-up questions about the thoughts, sensations, subjective feelings, and behavior or behavioral urges experienced. Such requests are then repeated approximately three more times over the course of the session, either in response to behavioral signs of increased anxiety (e.g., fidgeting, bouncing knee, furrowed brow) or during natural breaks in conversation while transitioning from one topic to another.

Within-session monitoring promotes the development of new self-monitoring habits from the outset of treatment. In addition, this procedure provides in-the-moment intervention opportunities during later sessions. For example, a therapist request for an anxiety rating during a cognitive therapy session might lead to identification of an automatic anxious thought that just occurred. This specific thought could then be challenged as the client experienced its immediate emotional impact, allowing cognitive restructuring of "hot" rather than "cold" cognition. Similarly, a therapist might notice visible muscle tension, bring this observation to the client's attention, and request an anxiety rating. As the client becomes aware of her excessive facial muscle tension, the therapist could suggest in-the-moment practice of progressive relaxation techniques. This repeated in-session practice teaches new coping responses to anxiety cues. Clients eventually practice these coping responses on their own as they detect anxiety cues between sessions.

## Self-Monitoring Homework Procedures

Early in treatment therapists present clients with a structured method for self-monitoring between sessions. Self-monitoring procedures involve either prepared forms with columns for anxiety ratings and other relevant information or step-by-step instructions for self-monitoring journal entries. Several published versions of prepared forms are currently available. These forms are briefly described below.

The *Mastery of your anxiety and worry, 2nd edition: Client workbook* (Craske & Barlow 2006a) presents clients with two self-monitoring forms to be completed throughout treatment. The Worry Record is a single-page form with five sets of ratings. Each time clients notice an increase in anxiety or bothersome worry, they record: the date, time, and duration of the episode, the maximum level of anxiety experienced on a 0–100 scale, any symptoms experienced, a brief description of any events that may have triggered the episode, anxious thoughts about feared outcomes or an inability to cope, and anxious behaviors. Clients are instructed to carry their Worry Records with them at all times so they can complete this form in the moment during each anxiety or worry episode.

The *Mastery of your anxiety and worry, 2nd edition: Client workbook* also instructs clients to complete a Daily Mood Record at the end of each day. This form contains columns for clients to record the date, overall anxiety rating for that day, maximum anxiety experienced during that day, overall physical tension, and overall preoccupation with worry. Barlow and colleagues also developed an alternative version of this form, the Weekly Record of Anxiety and Depression (WRAD; Brown, O'Leary, & Barlow 2001). In addition to average anxiety and maximum anxiety ratings, clients complete ratings of average depression, average pleasantness, and estimate the percentage of the day they felt worried.

In their GAD cognitive-behavior therapy manual, Rygh and Sanderson (2004) present their versions of these two types of self-monitoring forms. First, the Worry Diary instructs clients to make three estimates each day: percentage of the day spent in worry, overall level of anxiety rated with a 0–8 scale, and how many minutes were spent worrying that day. Clients also track their medication usage by recording the type of medication and the dosage taken. Second, clients complete the Worry Episode Log as worry episodes are noticed. Clients record the date and time of the episode, maximum intensity of anxiety experienced during the episode, amount of control over the episode, and ratings of any other emotions experienced such as anger or sadness. Internal and/or external triggers of the episode as well as thoughts and images, physical responses, and behavior identified during the episode are also noted. Finally, clients record how long the worry episode lasted.

Leahy and Holland (2000) created a single form, the Patient's Worry Log, to capture anxiety ratings as well as cognitive features of each worry. When worry is noticed, clients record the content, situational factors that bring out the worry, and specific predictions about what will happen. Clients then rate anxiety for each prediction as well as confidence in the accuracy of each prediction. Once the outcome has occurred, clients note the actual outcome and again rate their anxiety at the time of the outcome. Thus, this form prompts clients to monitor feared outcomes as they monitor their worry and anxiety from the beginning of treatment. A modified version of this form, the Worry Record, appears in the self-help book entitled *The worry cure* (Leahy 2005a). This Worry Record prompts readers to track the day and time of each worry, the events going on, how they felt right before the worry, the worry content, an anxiety rating, what they did next, and how they felt then. Readers are encouraged to review Worry Record entries, looking for patterns in the times, events, and behaviors most often associated with worry episodes.

A final form called the Worry Diary Form (Dugas & Robichaud 2007) is more streamlined, containing only four columns. Clients record the date and time a worry occurred, a brief description of the worry content, rating of current anxiety (on a 0–8 scale), and whether that worry represented a current problem or a hypothetical situation. The former type of worry is described as worry about a problem that already exists, while the latter type of worry concerns situations that have not actually happened and probably never will.

Although these forms vary in detail, some consistencies can be found across them. First, all require clients to rate their anxiety level on a frequent basis. Associated information, such as internal and external triggers, worry content or anxious thoughts noticed, and/or symptoms experienced, typically are included. Clients are instructed to complete forms either as anxiety or worry episodes are detected or at a pre-set regular time, such as the end of each day. Both versions of the Worry Record (Craske & Barlow 2006a and Leahy 2005a), the Worry Episode Log (Rygh & Sanderson 2004), the Patient's Worry Log (Leahy & Holland 2000), and the Worry Diary Form (Dugas & Robichaud 2007) all were designed to be filled out as clients notice episodes of high anxiety or worry. In contrast, the Daily Mood Record (Craske & Barlow 2006a), the Weekly Record of Anxiety and Depression (Brown et al. 2001), and the Worry Diary (Rygh & Sanderson 2004) are to be completed once per day regardless of how many episodes were experienced. Therapists often assign both types of monitoring to attain the benefits of each. Episodic forms provide objective information as anxiety and worry occurs, allowing clients to practice a new objective monitoring response to familiar anxiety cues. On the other hand, interval monitoring reminds clients to rate anxiety and reflect on their experience on a regular basis. This latter monitoring approach helps clients develop a new habit of checking in with oneself frequently to catch anxiety spirals as early as possible.

At our University of Nevada, Reno chronic worry intervention program, we combine these two monitoring approaches into a single form. Modeled after the Daily Diary developed by Borkovec and colleagues (Borkovec, Newman, Pincus, & Lytle 2002), clients check in and rate their current anxiety (on a 0–100 scale) at four pre-determined times each day. Instead of generating summary ratings at the end of each day, clients develop the habit of stopping their usual activity for a moment four times per day to rate how they feel at those specific points. Clients also record episodic information as they detect episodes of high anxiety. If a regularly scheduled anxiety rating is high (above 50) or if an anxiety episode reaching a peak of 50 or greater is detected between regular rating times, additional information about the episode is recorded in the lower portion of the form. Clients write down the circumstances surrounding the episode (including any internal and external triggers), a peak anxiety rating, and the individual anxiety components making up the anxiety spiral. Clients carry a copy of this form with them at all times to complete during the week. A copy of this Anxiety Diary Form and its written instructions are presented in Client Handout 4.1.

CLIENT HANDOUT 4.1.
_____
Anxiety diary form
_____

**Instructions:** Four times each day, check in and rate your current anxiety using the 0-100 scale shown below. Stop whatever you are doing for a moment to write down the time and to rate how you feel right at that moment. *Do not wait until the end of the day to record your ratings.* If your anxiety rating is 50 or higher, also write down the circumstances surrounding the episode (including any internal and external triggers), a peak anxiety rating, and the individual anxiety components making up the anxiety spiral in the lower portion of the form. If you notice an anxiety episode reaching a peak of 50 or greater between your regular rating times, record this information about the anxiety episode in the lower portion as well. Carry a copy of this form with you at all times to complete during the week.

```
           |----------------------------------+----------------------------------+
           0                                   50                               100
          No                               Moderate                          Severe
        Anxiety                             Anxiety                          Anxiety
Date & Day:     _____   _____   _____   _____   _____   _____   _____   _____

Waking up:      __/____    __/____    __/____    __/____    __/____    __/____    __/____    __/____

End of the
morning:        __/____    __/____    __/____    __/____    __/____    __/____    __/____    __/____

End of the
afternoon:      __/____    __/____    __/____    __/____    __/____    __/____    __/____    __/____

Bedtime:        __/____    __/____    __/____    __/____    __/____    __/____    __/____    __/____
```

If at any time, your anxiety grows to a level of 50 or greater, describe what was happening during that episode:

| Date/time | Circumstances and any thoughts, sensations, subjective feelings, and behavior or behavioral urges | Peak anxiety rating |
|-----------|----------------------------------------------------------------------|---------------------|
|           |                                                                      |                     |
|           |                                                                      |                     |
|           |                                                                      |                     |

Use the back of this sheet to record additional anxiety episodes.

In a self-help bibliotherapy intervention (Hazlett-Stevens 2005), clients receive step-by-step instructions to monitor their anxiety and worry in a note-book or journal. Rather than complete pre-printed forms, clients record essential information in their journal according to the same guidelines described above. Figure 4.1 contains this self-monitoring exercise, and a sample journal entry is presented in Fig. 4.2.

No available research has compared pre-printed monitoring forms to the journal approach. Prepared forms provide a standardized and consistent assessment method. Not surprisingly, the psychotherapy outcome investigations establishing empirical support for CBT utilized such prepared anxiety monitoring forms. In addition, pre-printed forms are designed to prompt client recording of all essen-tial information rather than rely on clients to remember which information to record on their own. However, because the journal entry method requires clients to generate all necessary information themselves, this method might foster quicker development of self-monitoring habits. Clients also might perceive the journal method as more individualized, thereby increasing a sense of personal accountability for self-monitor-ing. Regular self-monitoring becomes a new habit adopted to promote mental health and well-being instead of a stack of paperwork required by the therapist. Nevertheless, these apparent advantages and disadvantages are only speculative and have not been evaluated empirically.

## Self-Monitoring Homework Instructions

Regardless of the specific self-monitoring procedure or forms selected, thera-pists should review a set of guidelines to maximize client benefit. Therapists typically review the following instructions before regular self-monitoring at home begins:

1. Monitoring entries should be completed "on-the-spot" as the experience occurs. Recording information in the moment maximizes accuracy and fosters an objec-tive awareness of anxious experience as it happens. Retrospective reports are prone to memory biases and cognitive distortions.
2. Anxiety levels and subsequent reactions should be observed and recorded in an objective manner. Recorded entries only should contain concrete pieces of infor-mation such anxiety ratings, internal and external cues, and anxiety spiral thoughts, subjective feelings, bodily sensations, and behavior. Judgments about the experience or internal commentaries about perceived performance in the sit-uation are not included.
3. Monitoring entries must be done in writing. Clients most often need the practice and structure of writing this information down at first. Written records also allow clients to share this information with their therapists in subsequent sessions. Finally, previous self-monitoring data can be reviewed to assess therapy progress over the course of treatment.

1. Find a notepad and pencil or pen. Draw a horizontal line across the first page and write the number 0 on the left end and 100 on the right end. Put a hash mark in the middle and write the number 50 below it. It will look something like this:

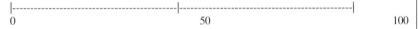

0                                                                      50                                                                    100

You'll use this simple scale to monitor your anxiety levels throughout this self-help program. Now try it for the first time. Ask yourself this question: If 100 is as anxious as I can possibly imagine, and 0 is completely and absolutely relaxed, how am I feeling right now? Of course there is no single "correct" answer to this question, but write down the number that best represents your current anxiety level. Put an exact number on your anxiety in the same sort of way your thermostat generates a number to indicate the current room temperature. This is the first step in looking at your anxiety and worry objectively.

2. Once you have come up with a number between 0 and 100 and written it down, ask yourself how you came up with it. Try to identify all you tuned into to arrive at that particular number. Underneath your anxiety rating, write down any thoughts you noticed. On the next line, list your subjective feelings. Then on the line underneath, jot down all bodily sensations. Finally, list any behaviors or movements you did or felt the urge to do. Be sure to list everything you notice that makes up your current experience. Here are some questions to ask:

- What were you just saying to yourself the split second before you came up with that rating?
- Were you having doubtful thoughts about whether this book can help you or whether you'll able to use it successfully?
- What subjective feelings did you notice? For example, were you feeling helpless, hopeless, frustrated, hopeful, or excited?
- Are certain muscles tense or relaxed?
- Are you sitting or breathing a certain way?
- Are you fidgeting or making any other anxiety-related movements?

Don't force yourself to decide what to include here—just write down everything you notice about your experience as matter-of-factly as you can.

3. Use the rest of your notepad as a diary to monitor your anxiety level several times a day, *every day*. Each page of your notebook can represent a different day. Each entry should begin with the time of day and a short description of what's happening around you, such as "sitting at my desk at work" or "just hung up the phone after talking to Mary." Then record a number between 0 and 100 to reflect your current anxiety rating and a description of whatever thoughts, feelings, sensations, and behaviors you noticed came up with that rating, exactly as you have just done in the previous steps. Remember to take time out throughout your day to make your diary entries—don't go back and write your entries after-the-fact from memory. Don't be tempted to skip the step of writing this down! Putting your entries in writing is part of what makes your monitoring objective. Plus, you'll be able to go back through your diary to track your progress, look for patterns, and learn what seems to trigger your worry. If you want even more practice to maximize your efforts, you can mentally monitor your anxiety by just thinking of a current rating. Do this in addition to the four to five times a day you make a written diary entry.

**Fig. 4.1** Self-monitoring journal exercise. Reprinted with permission from New Harbinger Publications, Inc., and Holly Hazlett-Stevens, *Women Who Worry Too Much: How to Stop Worry and Anxiety from Ruining Relationships, Work, and Fun*, Holly Hazlett-Stevens

Tuesday, Nov. 5th
  9:45 a.m.
  **Sitting at my desk**. My supervisor just asked for the project I'm still working on.
  **Anxiety rating:** 40
  **Thoughts:** How am I going to get this done before lunch? Why is my supervisor always so short with me? I hate this job.
  **Subjective feelings:** Frustrated and cranky—also still feeling sad from that dream last night.
  **Physical sensations:** My shoulders are tense and sore, butterflies and knots in my stomach, tightness in my upper chest.
  **Behaviors:** Biting my fingernails, tapping my pencil against my desk, feeling the urge to hide out in the bathroom for a few minutes.

**Fig. 4.2** Sample journal entry. Reprinted with permission from New Harbinger Publications, Inc., and Holly Hazlett-Stevens, *Women Who Worry Too Much: How to Stop Worry and Anxiety from Ruining Relationships, Work, and Fun*, Holly Hazlett-Stevens

4. Clients should set a schedule for self-monitoring ahead of time. Before the session ends, clients are encouraged to plan ahead and identify exactly when they will record their four anxiety ratings throughout each day. In addition, therapists clarify the criteria for high anxiety episodes and specify what information clients should record during each episode.
5. In addition to the self-monitoring written entries, therapists suggest even more frequent informal monitoring over the course of the day. Many external cues can serve as reminders to rate anxiety and identify any triggers and associated thoughts, sensations, feelings, and behavior. Clients can mentally practice such monitoring within a brief moment each time they remember. Common reminders can include every hour on the hour, each time the client begins a new task at work, each time the phone rings, or each time the client stops at a red light while driving. This informal practice promotes objective awareness of anxious experience and reinforces new self-monitoring habits.

## Chapter Summary

At the outset of CBT, therapists share essential information with clients to help them understand how therapy is expected to work and to increase their motivation to participate in treatment. During these initial psychoeducation sessions, therapists clarify any misconceptions about the GAD diagnosis and discuss background facts and statistics. Factors believed to contribute to the development of GAD are reviewed in light of the client's own family history and experiences. Cognitive-behavioral models of GAD as well as the avoidant function of worry are presented and discussed. Therapists then define terms such as fear, anxiety, and worry, explaining how some experience of each is a natural part of the human condition. Such "normal" experiences are compared to the excessive anxiety and worry associated with GAD and other anxiety disorders. Therapists also describe the different components of anxious experience and explain how anxious thoughts, sensations, subjective feelings, and behavior feed off each other in an "anxiety spiral." A rationale for treatment explains how relaxation training, cognitive restructuring, and behavioral interventions were designed to target each anxiety component, thereby interrupting automatic anxiety spirals. Regular and frequent objective monitoring of anxious experience provides the foundation for treatment, allowing clients to circumvent the development of anxiety spirals as early as possible. Finally, therapists make clients aware of the commitment involved in CBT. Therapists openly describe the time and effort required for successful behavior change, exploring any possible barriers that might be anticipated ahead of time. Although the psychoeducation treatment portion covers a substantial amount of new information, an interactive presentation style is preferred to a strictly didactic style whenever possible.

During initial therapy sessions, therapists also review the rationale and antici-pated benefits of anxiety monitoring. Therapists provide a structured method for the regular and frequent self-monitoring of anxiety levels, triggers, and anxiety spiral components. Several published forms are currently available, and our self-monitoring form developed at the University of Nevada, Reno is presented as Client Handout 4.1. This form combines a frequent interval monitoring approach with the anxiety episode self-monitoring approach. An alternative approach to self-monitoring uti-lizes client journal entries instead of pre-printed forms. This exercise is presented in Fig. 4.1 and was developed as part of a self-help bibliotherapy intervention (Hazlett-Stevens 2005), the effectiveness of which is still under empirical investigation. When instructing clients to self-monitor, therapists should emphasize that self-monitoring entries should be made on-the-spot rather than retrospectively and also should be recorded in writing. In addition to the written self-monitoring assignments, clients are encouraged to engage in informal self-monitoring at addi-tional times throughout the day. Therapists model this informal frequent anxiety monitoring by asking clients to rate their anxiety and identify associated thoughts, sensations, and behavior several times throughout each therapy session.

# Chapter 5
# Relaxation Strategies

Relaxation training benefits clients struggling with GAD in several ways. The ability to relax is a valuable life skill many clients did not learn naturally over the course of their development. Indeed, recent research has linked GAD symptoms to deficits in such fundamental emotion regulation abilities (Mennin, Heimberg, Turk, & Fresco 2005). In their emotion dysregulation model of GAD, Mennin and colleagues posited that heightened emotional intensity, fear of emotional experience, and poor ability to manage negative emotions characterize individuals with GAD (Mennin, Heimberg, Turk, & Fresco 2002; Mennin, Turk, Heimberg, & Carmin 2004). Maladaptive coping strategies such as unproductive worry result as individuals attempt to control physiological arousal and other facets of emotional experience. From this perspective, relaxation training teaches clients new and adaptive ways to manage, or even prevent, excessive physiological arousal and emotional reactivity. Anxiety spirals become less powerful when clients respond to early cues with relaxation coping responses in place of habitual anxiety-promoting reactions. Thus, relaxation training teaches clients new coping skills to apply during stressful situations or whenever anxiety cues are detected.

Relaxation practice also may reduce baseline levels of physiological arousal, particularly the central nervous system-mediated symptoms most often associated with GAD. Simply put, relaxation strategies directly target chronic anxiety symptoms such as muscle tension and physical restlessness. The more time spent in a state of relaxation instead of somatic anxiety, the less likely anxiety spirals will develop in the first place. Perceptions of threat and worry also are less likely to occur while relaxed than while tense. For this reason, therapists often describe relaxation as a new set of habits and a lifestyle change that clients can adopt indefinitely. Furthermore, continued relaxation practice might alleviate any associated physical complaints, such as irritable bowel syndrome (IBS) or other gastrointestinal distress, headaches, or chronic neck and back pain.

The present-moment focus of attention inherent in relaxation practice has received increasing interest in recent years. Relaxation training requires clients to concentrate on physical sensations, body movements, and internal experiences as they occur. This attentional focus on the present moment is essentially incompatible with the future-oriented thinking that characterizes worry. Borkovec (2002) suggested that GAD clients miss essential information provided in the present

H. Hazlett-Stevens, *Psychological Approaches to Generalized Anxiety Disorder,*
doi: 10.1007/978-0-387-76870-0, © Springer Science+Business Media, LLC 2008

moment because they devote their attentional resources to worry about possible future outcomes. Thus, useful information from the immediate environment as well as primary emotional experience is not processed and therefore cannot motivate or guide behavior in adaptive ways. Relaxation training might be of particular benefit to GAD clients because relaxation skills involve mental focus on the present moment and redirection of attention back to the present when distracted.

Not surprisingly, clinicians often emphasize this present-moment-focus aspect of relaxation training when treating GAD. For example, therapists provide explicit instructions and procedures that help clients practice present-moment focus during formal relaxation practice. Therapists also encourage clients to redirect their attention back to the present moment whenever a worry is detected and postponed. Such clinical practice is quite consistent with "mindfulness" therapy procedures. During mindfulness exercises, clients practice observing present-moment internal experience in a nonjudgmental, open, and compassionate fashion. Clients also might practice mindfulness outside of therapy sessions in yoga or meditation classes. Consistent with outcome research demonstrating the effectiveness of a Mindfulness-Based Stress Reduction (MBSR) intervention (Kabat-Zinn, Massion, Kristeller, Peterson, et al. 1992; Miller, Fletcher, & Kabat-Zinn 1995), Roemer and Orsillo (2005) have integrated mindfulness into the diaphragmatic breathing and progressive relaxation components of their acceptance-based behavior therapy for GAD.

Some experts have expressed concern that relaxation training may be counter-productive (e.g., Hayes, Strosahl, & Wilson 1999). Teaching clients to relax may inadvertently suggest that anxious arousal is harmful, should not be experienced, and therefore needs to be controlled, in direct contradiction to the psychoeducation information presented earlier. On a related note, exposure to feared internal and external stimuli is vital to the effective treatment of anxiety disorders. In addition to external situations and outcomes, GAD clients often fear the bodily sensations associated with anxious arousal. For exposure to be effective, clients must face their feared situations or scenarios with the associated subjective experience of fear and anxiety-related physiology. Thus, client attempts to control or avoid unwanted physiology with relaxation skills could undermine the exposure exercises described in Chap. 7. Furthermore, such attempts typically fail to reduce unwanted physiology. Many clinicians have observed the quintessential paradox of relaxation training: the harder a client tries to relax, the more elusive relaxation becomes. As clients desperately try to avoid anxious experience with relaxation skills, they become less likely to experience skill mastery or to perceive treatment as useful.

One possible response to this concern is to eliminate relaxation training altogether. However, this option leaves clients without an essential emotion regulation coping skill. Alternatively, therapists might discuss this potential pitfall with clients at the outset of relaxation training. Relaxation skills are best considered a method for coping with difficult situations rather than a way of escaping discomfort. When clients encounter daily life situations in a relaxed state, they are better able to view events objectively and therefore respond effectively. On the other hand, anxious arousal is inevitable and sometimes even useful. During exposure exercises, clients will practice tolerating fear and anxiety as they confront difficult situations and images. In fact, clients will be instructed to allow and to experience fully the emotional reactions they previously resisted. Thus, coping with anxiety is best conceptualized as a dialectical process. Indeed, experts in the treatment of other psychological disorders associated with emotion regulation deficits have emphasized the importance of both types of skills (Fruzzetti, Shenk, Mosco, & Lowry 2003; Linehan 1993). Acceptance skills are designed to help individuals accept their emotions, whereas change skills involve altering emotions. Clients can learn to tolerate discomfort and act effectively while anxious. At the same time, they can develop skills to modulate subjective reactions, physiological arousal, and anxiety-provoking thoughts in the service of promoting effective behavior.

Three separate relaxation strategies are particularly useful for clients with GAD. First, deep breathing exercises teach clients to breathe from the diaphragm muscle located in the abdomen. Most clients have developed automatic habits of shallow chest breathing at an accelerated rate. Physical sensations resembling anxiety symptoms naturally result from this subtle hyperventilation over time, due to the imbalance of oxygen and carbon dioxide in the blood associated with overbreathing. This relaxation strategy targets the cumulative effects of shallow and fast breathing habits by teaching clients to shift to slow and deep breathing whenever useful. Second, progressive relaxation training targets chronic muscle tension. Clients begin by tensing and releasing 16 isolated muscle groups in formal practice sessions, combining these into fewer muscle groups in subsequent practice sessions. Clients eventually learn to identify unnecessary muscle tension at other times during the day and are able to relax specific muscles whenever such tension is detected. Finally, clients practice relaxation through mental imagery. Clients learn to create vivid images that generate feelings of relaxation with the goal of visualizing these relaxing scenes at useful times during the day. As clients develop each of these relaxation skills, therapists encourage them to apply these skills as they encounter anxiety cues and stressful situations. Clients learn and practice all three strategies to provide multiple options for responding and to increase response flexibility. Ideally, clients will experiment with the deployment of different relaxation responses at different times and will discover which strategies work best for them in certain contexts.

Relaxation training requires daily formal practice to build necessary skills. Therapists demonstrate relaxation procedures during sessions, but clients must follow through with home practice. Clients also will incorporate brief relaxation practices into their daily routine once their relaxation skills have developed with formal practice. Thus, effective relaxation training involves many home practice assignments, requiring much effort and dedication from clients. For this reason, some therapists ask clients to keep a written record of their relaxation practice each week. Therapists can create a home practice log form with columns for the date and time of each practice, length of practice, description of what was practiced, and how the practice was experienced. This form either can be assigned to clients from the beginning or after clients report difficulty following through with planned practice. Tracking completed home practice assignments might increase compliance and hold clients accountable for their practice. However, some clients may view home practice log forms as an additional burden or perceive the therapist as overly paternalistic for assigning them. Furthermore, client reports of practice do not necessarily reflect the amount of actual practice that occurred. Clients may over-report their practice to avoid embarrassment or disapproval. Regardless of whether or not therapists ask clients to record their practice, therapists should discuss home practice with their clients in a fashion that fosters a collaborative therapeutic relationship.

## Diaphragmatic Breathing

Deep breathing relaxation, also known as diaphragmatic breathing or breathing retraining, is easy to teach in a short period of time. Therapists often present this relaxation technique first, immediately after psychoeducation and anxiety monitoring topics are covered. Therapists might demonstrate diaphragmatic breathing and assign home practice as early as the first session, giving clients an opportunity to engage in new behavior from the outset of treatment. This intervention begins with a brief rationale. Next, the therapist demonstrates shallow chest breathing and deep diaphragmatic stomach breathing. As the client attempts deep breathing, the therapist observes and gives specific feedback until the client is effectively breathing from the abdomen at a slow and regular rate. Finally, the therapist introduces a present-moment focus component in which the client redirects attention back to the breathing practice each time the mind wanders off. Daily formal home practice continues until the client routinely applies this relaxation skill in daily life.

### *Diaphragmatic Breathing Rationale*

Therapists explain this relaxation technique by drawing a contrast between two different ways of breathing. In the first, breathing takes place in the abdomen. Each breath involves a large curved abdominal muscle called the diaphragm, so the stomach rises and falls with each breath without using the chest muscles much at all. This first type of breathing, diaphragmatic breathing, reflects how our bodies are designed to breathe. Has the client ever noticed the breathing patterns of someone sleeping soundly on his or her back? Each breath involves a slow, fluid, continuous motion that begins low in the abdomen. The stomach fully expands with each inhalation and then falls with each exhalation. Diaphragmatic breathing might generate physical sensations of relaxation by stimulating the parasympathetic branch of the autonomic nervous system. This part of the nervous system slows the body down, allowing for digestion to occur as the body rests. Diaphragmatic breathing also might optimize blood oxygen levels, thereby preventing the anxiety-like sensations associated with an imbalance of oxygen and carbon dioxide. Finally, deep breathing practice creates subjective feelings of relaxation as clients become increasingly comfortable with various bodily sensations.

During times of stress, the diaphragm muscle contracts. The lungs themselves do not have muscles, so the body automatically relies upon the nearby chest muscles to do the work of breathing. However, chest muscles did not evolve for the purpose of breathing as the diaphragm muscle did. Therefore, this second way of breathing from the chest is more shallow and uncomfortable than natural diaphragmatic breathing. Chest muscles often become sore from overuse. Breathing becomes faster than necessary to meet the body's needs, causing subtle hyperventilation effects that build over time. Furthermore, shallow and rapid chest breathing stimulates the sympathetic branch of the autonomic nervous system. This particular physiological effect produces many of the same arousal sensations that are experienced during times of anxiety. In short, diaphragmatic breathing creates a physical state of relaxation whereas shallow chest breathing creates physiological arousal and anxiety-like sensations which often lead to subjective anxiety.

Most people have developed habitual ways of breathing. Because constant breathing is essential to our survival, we can breathe automatically without any effort or conscious awareness. However, with a little effort we also can exert control over our breathing and therefore develop new and adaptive breathing habits. Most people habitually breathe from some combination of the chest and the abdomen. Individuals prone to anxiety typically engage in more chest breathing than diaphragmatic breathing. The purpose of diaphragmatic breathing is to breathe in an optimal way as much of the time as possible. Formal practice teaches clients to exert voluntary control over breathing patterns. Eventually clients will develop new diaphragmatic breathing habits and will practice voluntary shifting to deep diaphragmatic breathing whenever old chest breathing patterns are detected.

## *Diaphragmatic Breathing Session Procedures*

Once the client understands the basic rationale behind diaphragmatic breathing, the therapist demonstrates chest breathing and diaphragmatic abdominal breathing. The therapist puts one hand on his or her chest and the other hand on his or her stomach. The therapist then invites the client to observe how both hands move, evidence that the therapist is breathing from both the chest and the stomach. Next, the therapist purposefully isolates breathing to the chest and asks the client to notice how only the top hand is moving. This brief demonstration concludes with the therapist shifting to the desired deep diaphragmatic breathing in which only the bottom hand moves.

After this demonstration, the therapist asks the client to try the same. The client puts one hand on his or her chest and the other hand on his or her stomach while continuing to breathe normally. The therapist points out how much of the client's habitual breathing patterns involve chest breathing as both the client and therapist observe which hand(s) are moving. Next, the therapist asks the client to isolate breathing from the stomach such that only the bottom hand moves while the top hand on the chest remains still. Ideally the client breathes completely through the nose, although keeping the mouth closed might not be feasible due to nasal congestion or other physical factors. As the client attempts diaphragmatic breathing, the therapist closely observes while providing encouragement and feedback. Oftentimes, the client will incorporate more of the abdomen than his or her initial breathing but still exhibit some breathing from the chest. In this case, simply pointing out that the top hand is still moving slightly and encouraging the client to breathe from the stomach even deeper will suffice.

If the client experiences difficulty isolating the abdomen, the therapist can suggest relaxing the abdominal muscles as completely as possible while purposefully expanding the abdomen a bit just before each inhalation. The client also might benefit from instructions to keep the chest and shoulders as still as possible while breathing. Some therapists ask clients to close their eyes and imagine a large balloon in their abdomen filling with air during each inhalation and deflating with each exhalation. If these quick tips are not effective, the client could lie flat on the floor or a firm couch on his or her stomach (i.e., face-down) with both hands clasped under the forehead. Once the client begins to breathe from the abdomen in this position, he or she moves back to a seated position while continuing to breathe with the diaphragm.

Clients exhibiting rapid, shallow, or erratic breathing patterns may experience some difficulty at first. These clients may report that diaphragmatic breathing seems artificial or that they feel even more breathless or anxious instead of relaxed. Therapists can reassure clients that such sensations are not harmful and that such a reaction is not surprising, given how dramatically this way of breathing differs from their usual way. These clients may need to spend a few extra minutes attempting diaphragmatic breathing with therapist feedback and encouragement. Therapist comments that many people find diaphragmatic breathing difficult to learn and that clients often report the experience as strange, unfamiliar, and even uncomfortable at first can help normalize client reactions.

After the client has successfully isolated breathing to the diaphragm, the therapist instructs the client to slow the rate of breathing to 8–10 breaths per minute. This rate allows approximately 3–4 seconds for each inhalation and 3–4 seconds per exhalation. Slow diaphragmatic breathing also should be smooth and fluid. The therapist therefore guides the client toward continuous air flow and easy breathing movements rather than abrupt or erratic breathing patterns. Instruction to allow the air to escape equally over the entire exhalation instead of suddenly releasing it might be helpful. Furthermore, the client should not hold his or her breath during diaphragmatic breathing practice, nor should the client feel as if he or she is gasping for air.

Now that the client has learned to breathe from the diaphragm correctly, the therapist introduces a mental present-moment focus component. For some clients, instructions to keep the mind focused on the physical sensations of deep breathing while gently bringing the mind back to these sensations whenever it wanders are most effective. We have experimented with this mindfulness present-moment focus task at our University of Nevada, Reno chronic worry intervention program. Clients are asked to focus all of their attention on breathing sensations, noticing how the air feels as it enters the body and moves down into the abdomen which expands with each inhalation. Likewise, clients fully experience the physical sensations of each exhalation as the stomach begins to fall and the air slowly escapes through the nose and/or mouth. As the mind wanders from these breathing sensations, clients practice gently bringing their full awareness back to the breath. Clients regard any thoughts, feelings, or other experiences as streams of events passing through the mind rather than reacting to them.

Clients familiar with the term "mindfulness" who have practiced this skill before in yoga or meditation classes might prefer this approach. Therapists often present "mindfulness" as a special way of experiencing the present moment. In addition to focusing attention on the present, mindfulness practice involves allowing oneself to experiencing all aspects of each moment in an accepting way. An attitude of patience and freedom from judging certain thoughts, feelings, and sensations as good or bad are cultivated during mindfulness practice. Jon Kabat-Zinn (1994) offered the following popular definition of mindfulness:

> Mindfulness means paying attention in a particular way: on purpose, in the present moment, and nonjudgmentally. This kind of attention nurtures greater awareness, clarity, and acceptance of present-moment reality. (p. 4)

Other clients may express skepticism of mindfulness practice or meditation procedures. These clients tend to benefit from a structured mental focus task during diaphragmatic breathing practice instead. One possible task (Barlow & Craske 2006; Craske & Barlow 2006b) involves silently counting each breath during inhalation, then thinking a word such as "relax" or "calm" to oneself with each exhalation. Each inhalation is counted up to ten, then back down to one, again up to ten, and so on for the duration of the practice session. A variation on this mental task (Rygh & Sanderson 2004) involves covertly repeating the word "relax" with each breath. The client thinks the syllable "re" during each inhalation and the syllable "lax" during each exhalation. Similar to mindfulness practice instructions, clients are asked to notice and let go of any distracting thoughts or images as they occur. Clients then re-focus their attention on the mental task at hand. Therapists should make sure clients expect present-moment focus to be challenging at first. Clients should be aware that "perfect" performance on this task is nearly impossible, as human minds naturally tend to wander. Therapists encourage clients to view each time the mind wanders as an opportunity to practice re-focusing attention on the present moment rather than feeling discouraged and giving up.

Some therapists ask each client to try the mindfulness instructions for a few minutes and evaluate client response in session. These therapists introduce the structured mental tasks described above (e.g., counting breaths or repeating the word "re-lax") only if a client experiences significant difficulty keeping the mind focused on breathing sensations. Structured mental focus tasks also might be beneficial when a client appears resistant to mindfulness practice or in need of a specific internal stimulus to focus attention. In a second approach, therapists start each client with either the breath counting or the "re-lax" mental focus task. Mindfulness practice instructions are introduced a few sessions later, after clients have mastered a structured present-moment focus task. In a final method, therapists invite clients to try each present-moment focus task in session and select the one that seems to works best for them. In later sessions, clients are encouraged to try the other mental focus tasks once the practiced task becomes familiar. Therapists may opt for this third approach to model flexibility for clients. Clients learn different ways to practice present-moment focus with the goal of personal experimentation. This intervention strategy reflects the collaborative empiricism concept central to CBT. In addition, therapeutic alliance is often strengthened when clients feel they have choices and that their therapist values their input when making treatment decisions.

## Optional Alternative Procedure for Panic Symptoms

An alternative way of presenting this breathing technique may be helpful to clients with comorbid panic disorder or complaints of recurrent panic attacks. Craske and Barlow (2006b) recommended that therapists ask clients with panic disorder to hyperventilate before explaining the breathing retraining rationale. Clients experience the physical effects of hyperventilation first-hand just before therapists discuss the physiology involved. This clinical practice demonstrates that dramatic panic-related sensations can be elicited voluntarily and are not physically dangerous. Clients are more likely to appreciate the link between rapid shallow breathing and associated physical sensations if they have just produced these sensations in session.

Therapists ask clients to stand and to hyperventilate by breathing hard and fast as if they are blowing up a balloon. Exhalations should be forced and approximately three times the normal rate. Therapists usually demonstrate hyperventilation for a few breaths first and often hyperventilate with the client for much of the time. After 60–90 seconds of purposeful hyperventilation, sooner in cases of extreme distress, therapists ask clients to sit down, try to relax, and breathe slowly and comfortably. Clients are invited to describe the sensations experienced and to compare these sensations to their panic and anxiety symptoms. Therapists then present the diaphragmatic breathing rationale and explain the physiology that occurs during hyperventilation, followed by the same procedures described above (i.e., therapist demonstration of diaphragmatic breathing, client practice of slow and deep stomach breathing with therapist feedback, and introduction of a present-moment mental component). Clients read additional psychoeducation information about the physiological changes associated with hyperventilation. For further information about this optional procedure, the reader is referred to *Mastery of your anxiety and panic, 4th edition* (MAP-4) Client Workbook (Barlow & Craske 2006) and Therapist Guide (Craske & Barlow 2006b) and Hazlett-Stevens and Craske (2003a).

## Diaphragmatic Breathing Home Practice

The initial diaphragmatic breathing training session should conclude with assignment of formal home practice. Clients develop this relaxation skill from scheduled daily practice sessions that take place in a calm setting free from distractions. The following instructions are reviewed with clients before they begin their formal home practice:

1. Set aside two times per day, at least 10 min each, when you can devote all your time and attention to breathing practice. Conduct each practice in a quiet and comfortable place where you will not be disturbed. Make any necessary arrangements ahead of time, such as asking others in your home not to disturb you, turning off the telephone ringer and television, or making a trip to the bathroom. If you are concerned about losing track of time during your practice sessions because you have something else scheduled soon afterward, set a timer or alarm clock.
2. Loosen any tight clothing and remove your watch, jewelry, shoes, eyeglasses, and anything else that creates pressure on your body.
3. Begin each practice session by giving yourself a few seconds to calm down after closing your eyes. Place one hand on your chest and the other hand on your stomach, just as we have done here, and shift your breathing all the way down to your stomach until only your bottom hand moves. Once you have achieved deep diaphragmatic breathing, slow your breathing rate down to 8–10 breathing cycles per minute. Make sure that your breathing pattern is smooth and fluid, with continuous and even air flow throughout each inhalation and each exhalation.
4. Begin the present-moment focus component, either by directing all your attention to the physical sensations of breathing, by silently counting each inhalation and thinking "relax" or a similar word with each exhalation, or by thinking "re" while inhaling and "lax" while exhaling. As you notice your mind wandering away from the present moment, gently bring it back to the sensations of breathing and/or the present-moment focus task. Continue this formal practice for the full 10 min.

In addition to these formal home practice sessions, therapists also encourage clients to apply this new skill over the course of the day. When clients detect increases in anxiety through self-monitoring, they can respond with slow and deep diaphragmatic breathing. Clients should try to make this new way of breathing a constant habit by shifting to diaphragmatic breathing each time they notice they have reverted back to chest breathing. This combination of formal home practice for skill development and application of this relaxation skill in daily life will help clients develop new diaphragmatic breathing habits. Eventually this preferred way of breathing will become automatic, replacing current shallow chest breathing habits. Later in treatment, this relaxation strategy will be incorporated into additional applied relaxation procedures over the course of the day.

In each subsequent therapy session, therapists follow up with clients by asking about their experience with formal and applied diaphragmatic breathing practice. Often therapists will ask clients to engage in diaphragmatic breathing during the subsequent session. Therapists then make sure clients are breathing correctly and give encouragement and, if necessary, any corrective feedback. Any reported difficulties following through with scheduled practice can be addressed as well. After clients report two full weeks of twice daily formal practice, therapists might suggest eliminating one or both formal practice sessions. Clients are then encouraged to engage in diaphragmatic breathing as much as possible throughout each day. However, by this time many clients report that formal practice sessions have become a welcome routine. Formal diaphragmatic breathing practice with the present-moment focus component offers a retreat from daily life that ultimately allows clients to function more effectively during the rest of the day.

## Progressive Relaxation Training

Progressive relaxation, sometimes referred to as progressive muscle relaxation, dates back to the 1930's. Physiologist Edmund Jacobson observed that the physical muscle tension arising from shortened, contracted muscle fibers was associated with complaints of anxiety. He also viewed relaxation of muscle fibers to be the exact opposite physiological state. Jacobson therefore proposed that anxious individuals might benefit from learning to relax and elongate their muscles. If such individuals could learn to create an opposing physiology to their typical muscle tension physiology, then perhaps psychological states of anxiety would be alleviated. Jacobson soon developed an elaborate system for tensing and releasing dozens of muscle groups. Individuals purposefully tensed and released tension of isolated muscles while paying careful attention to associated physical sensations. Individuals learned to discriminate sensations of muscle contraction from complete relaxation with the eventual goal of detecting and releasing even the slightest degree of unnecessary muscle tension. Jacobson first described this relaxation technique for the general public in 1934. A few years later, in 1938, he documented these procedures for clinicians in his seminal book, *Progressive relaxation*. By the 1960's Jacobson had streamlined his original progressive relaxation technique to only 15 muscle groups, but his training program typically lasted for 56 sessions and sometimes much longer.

Joseph Wolpe is most widely recognized for his systematic desensitization procedure, an exposure-based behavior therapy for specific fears and phobias (1958). During the development of this therapy procedure, Wolpe searched for a way of inducing a physiological state incompatible with fear and anxiety. He considered Jacobson's progressive relaxation a promising technique but found the length of time required to implement it impractical. Wolpe therefore reduced Jacobson's original procedures to six therapy sessions with two home practice sessions per day. Thus, Wolpe is credited as the first behavior therapist to shorten Jacobsonian progressive relaxation training substantially. His efforts resulted in a convenient and practical relaxation procedure that could be implemented in a variety of clinical settings.

In the 1970's clinical psychologists Douglas Bernstein and Thomas Borkovec developed a structured abbreviated progressive relaxation training (PRT) program. Their 10-session protocol involved teaching clients to tense and release 16 different muscle groups systematically in session followed by twice daily formal practice sessions. Once clients mastered this procedure, subsequent PRT sessions combined muscle groups down to seven and eventually only four. Further reduction in the time needed to achieve deep muscle relaxation was accomplished with recall procedures. Clients practiced focusing attention on each of the 4 muscle groups to detect any tension. While recalling sensations associated with tension release in those muscles, clients were instructed to relax away any residual muscle tension. Clients also practiced this procedure with counting, achieving a deeper state of relaxation with each number counted. Eventually clients could attain a deep state of relaxation within 1 min by counting alone. Since the publication of their 1973 manual, this abbreviated PRT has been widely studied. PRT has received empirical support, either alone or as a component of a larger treatment package, for numerous anxiety and behavioral medicine conditions including GAD (see Bernstein, Borkovec, &

Hazlett-Stevens 2000 for a review of this literature). The PRT procedures described below are based on the updated manual by Bernstein and colleagues (2000) entitled *New directions in progressive relaxation training*.

## *Progressive Relaxation Training Rationale*

PRT teaches GAD clients how to reduce chronic tension. From a theoretical perspective, the excessive muscle tension associated with GAD contributes to the development of anxiety spirals. PRT targets this somatic component of anxiety spirals directly. Thus, one purpose of PRT is to reduce baseline levels of muscle tension. Repeated practice sessions teach clients to detect and reduce unnecessary muscle tension. In addition, this practice requires present-moment focus on bodily sensations. Finally, PRT skills eventually can be applied as a coping response to stressful situations and anxiety spiral triggers.

After explaining the role of muscle tension in GAD and why PRT may be a useful treatment approach, therapists typically cover additional rationale material specific to the PRT technique. Bernstein et al. (2000) presented a standard rationale that informs clients about the nature of PRT and the reasoning behind specific procedures. This rationale begins with a brief description of the history behind PRT. Therapists then explain the basic procedure in which clients learn to tense and relax isolated muscle groups in a systematic fashion. Tension and release cycles are conducted with careful attention to accompanying physical sensations so that clients learn to identify specific sources of excess muscle tension as they occur. The importance of home practice for skill development is emphasized. In addition, therapists explain the advantages of first producing tension before relaxing each muscle group. Clients are better able to study muscle tension sensations when they purposefully create noticeable levels of muscle tension. This tension-release procedure also creates a momentum, resulting in greater muscle relaxation than if clients simply relaxed a muscle group from its natural resting state. An outline of the PRT rationale content recommended by Bernstein et al. (2000) appears in Fig. 5.1.

---

A. The procedures to be used are called progressive relaxation training.

B. Progressive relaxation training consists of learning to tense and release various muscle groups throughout the body.

C. An essential part of learning how to relax involves learning to pay close attention to the feelings of tension and relaxation in your body.

D. Learning relaxation skills is like learning other motor skills. (I will not be doing anything to you; you will simply be learning a technique.)

E. We employ tension in order to ultimately produce relaxation.

1. Strong tension is noticeable and you will learn to attend to these feelings.

2. The initial production of tension gives us some "momentum" so that when we release the tension deep relaxation is the result.

F. Questions and comments.

---

**Fig. 5.1** PRT Rationale Content Outline. *New Directions in Progressive Relaxation Training: A Guidebook for Helping Professionals*, Bernstein, Borkovec, and Hazlett-Stevens (2000). Copyright © 2000 by Douglas. A. Bernstein and Thomas D. Borkovec. Reproduced with permission of Greenwood Publishing Group, Inc., Westport, CT.

## *Initial Progressive Relaxation Training Session Procedures*

Immediately after PRT rationale presentation, therapists demonstrate how to tense and relax each of 16 isolated muscle groups. Therapists follow the same format for each of the 16 muscle groups: (1) ask clients to tense the specific muscle group, (2) give explicit instructions for producing tension in that muscle group, (3) show clients how tension is accomplished, (4) make sure clients feel tension in the appropriate muscles before relaxing, and (5) move on to the next muscle group. Therapists might provide additional support and encouragement when asking clients to tense the muscles of the face, as some clients feel embarrassed by their resulting facial expressions. Therapist modeling of facial muscle tension before asking clients to do so might help reassure clients. Therapists also can acknowledge that this procedure might seem strange because it involves making funny faces. When demonstrating tension in the calves and feet, therapists should ask clients to tense for only a few seconds each time to prevent muscle cramping. The 16 muscle groups and specific instructions for producing tension in each provided by Bernstein et al. (2000) are reprinted in Fig. 5.2.

---

A.  We will be dealing with 16 muscle groups which are tensed and released. As skill develops, the number of groups will be reduced
B.  Tensing instructions for arms and hands (Determine which side is dominant.)
    1. Instructions for dominant hand and lower arm (Make tight fist.)
    2. Instructions for dominant biceps (Push elbow down against chair.)
    3. Instructions for nondominant hand and lower arm
    4. Instructions for nondominant biceps
C.  Tensing instructions for face and neck (Model face-making to put client at ease.)
    1. Instructions for forehead (Lift eyebrows as high as possible.)
    2. Instructions for central section (Squint and wrinkle nose.)
    3. Instructions for lower face and jaw (Bite hard and pull back corners of mouth.)
    4. Instructions for neck (Pull chin toward chest and keep it from touching chest.)
D.  Tensing instructions for chest and abdomen
    1. Instructions for chest, shoulders, and upper back (Pull shoulder blades together.)
    2. Instructions for abdomen (Make stomach hard.)
E.  Tensing instructions for legs and feet
    1. Instructions for dominant upper leg (Counterpose top and bottom muscles.)
    2. Instructions for dominant calf (Pull toes toward head.)
    3. Instructions for dominant foot (Point and curl toes, turning foot inward.)
    4. Instructions for nondominant upper leg
    5. Instructions for nondominant calf
    6. Instructions for nondominant foot
F.  Questions and comments (Be sure alternative tensing strategies are determined where needed.)

---

**Fig. 5.2** Tensing Instructions. *New Directions in Progressive Relaxation Training: A Guidebook for Helping Professionals*, Bernstein, Borkovec, and Hazlett-Stevens (2000). Copyright © 2000 by Douglas. A. Bernstein and Thomas D. Borkovec. Reproduced with permission of Greenwood Publishing Group, Inc., Westport, CT.

Once clients understand how to produce tension in each muscle group, therapists guide clients through their first formal practice session. At this time, therapists often ask clients to rate their current anxiety. This pre-relaxation rating allows clients to evaluate the immediate effects of the relaxation procedure in an objective way. Clients are encouraged to rate their anxiety just before and immediately following each home practice session as well. Clients track their relaxation training progress by recording each rating in their self-monitoring forms. This method serves an additional function of providing therapists a written record of home practice frequency.

Some experts discourage audiotaping in-session relaxation training practice out of concern that clients will depend upon the audiotape for home practice. The ultimate goal of PRT is identification and immediate release of excess muscle tension in any setting. Clients therefore should learn to create and to release tension in each isolated muscle group on their own as soon as possible. However, clients often report initial difficulty remembering the sequence of the muscle groups and how to produce tension in each. Clients also find that timing the tension and release cycles (e.g., 5–7 seconds of tension, 30–40 seconds of relaxation) distracts their attention away from the present moment and associated physical sensations during the practice session. For this reason, therapists can audiotape the therapist-guided procedure in session but instruct clients to use the audiotape only during the first few home practice sessions. Once clients have learned the procedure, their home practice sessions continue without the tape.

The in-session procedures developed by Bernstein and Borkovec are summarized here and are presented in greater detail in their updated PRT manual (Bernstein et al. 2000). Therapists create a relaxing setting for clients by reducing outside noise and distractions as much as possible, dimming the lights, and providing clients with a comfortable chair that completely supports their body weight. Similar to home practice instructions, clients are asked to loosen any tight clothing and to remove any watches, jewelry, eyeglasses, and shoes.

Therapists begin this formal practice by inviting clients to close their eyes, to settle into the chair, and to notice the sensations of their body touching the chair. Following the same sequence as the muscle tension demonstration, therapists ask clients to focus all their attention on the muscles of the first muscle group (i.e., right hand and forearm). Next, therapists instruct clients to produce tension in those muscles, reminding them of specific tension instructions for that muscle group. Therapists should clearly state when clients are expected to create the tension with a cue word or phrase such as "right now." Clients hold the tension while studying associated sensations for approximately 5–7 seconds. Therapists then instruct clients to release all tension immediately with a clear statement such as "And now, relax." Clients focus all attention on the sensations of muscle relaxation for the next 30–40 seconds. During this time, therapists paraphrase directions to notice sensations of relaxation in these muscles and compare relaxation sensations with previously produced tension sensations. Such relaxation training "patter" should encourage present-moment focus on the bodily sensations felt in that specific muscle group and should not contain hypnotic suggestions for how clients are feeling or should be feeling. Some therapists integrate mindfulness instructions into their relaxation patter by encouraging clients to bring attention back to current sensations in specific muscles whenever they notice the mind has wandered. A sample transcript portraying what therapists might say as they guide clients through the first cycle of the first muscle group appears below. Additional relaxation patter suggestions appear in Bernstein et al. (2000). Therapists should speak in a smooth and conversational tone, pausing between phrases.

> Therapist: Begin by focusing all your attention on the muscles of your right hand and forearm...and tense these muscles, making a tight fist, right now...notice what tension feels like in these muscles...feel them pulling in the fingers, over the top of the knuckles, across the wrist, and all through the lower arm...and now, relax...let all the tension go...notice how different these muscles feel now that they're completely relaxed...how different these feelings of relaxation are from the tension just produced...feel these muscles relaxing more and more deeply...savoring feelings of relaxation as these muscles smooth out and unwind...bringing the mind back if it has wandered...back to these muscles, noticing how relaxed and loose they feel...nothing to do but relax...

The tension-release cycle is then repeated for the first muscle group. Clients again are asked to tense only those muscles with specific tension-producing instructions. After 5–7 seconds concentrating on associated tension sensations, clients release the tension and focus on relaxation sensations. Relaxation typically follows for 45–60 seconds the second time to help clients achieve deep muscle relaxation before moving on to the next muscle group. After approximately 45 seconds have elapsed, therapists ask clients to signal when those muscles feel completely relaxed by lifting a finger. Therapists then proceed to the second muscle group and guide clients through two tension-release cycles for that muscle group. The PRT practice session continues in this way until clients have completed two cycles for each subsequent muscle group. At the end of the second cycle for each subsequent muscle group, clients are instructed to signal when the muscles of the current group are as relaxed as the previous muscle group. To prevent cramping of muscle groups involving the lower legs and feet, therapists should instruct clients to hold the tension in these muscles for only 3–4 seconds.

After two cycles of each muscle group, ideally after clients have signaled deep relaxation in each, therapists review each muscle group and instruct clients to allow each to continue relaxing. To ensure that clients are as relaxed as possible, therapists can ask clients to signal if they feel even the slightest bit of tension anywhere in the body. If clients do signal, therapists list the different muscle groups and ask clients to signal when the muscle group with tension is named. Therapists then instruct clients to tense those muscles again followed by complete release of any residual tension. Finally, therapists ask clients to signal when they feel completely relaxed throughout the entire body. After this signal, clients are invited to enjoy this state of complete relaxation for a few minutes more.

This relaxation training session is terminated by therapists counting backward from four to one. Therapists ask clients to move the legs and feet on the count of four, to move the arms and hands on the count of three, and to move the head and neck on the count of two. At the count of one, clients are invited to open their eyes whenever they are ready to resume the therapy session. After audiotape recording has ended, clients provide a post-relaxation anxiety rating and therapists ask clients about their experience. Therapists might acknowledge that coming out of a deeply relaxed state can feel disorienting or similar to waking up from sleep. Open-ended questions about subjective feelings of relaxation as well as pointed questions about which muscle groups were most difficult to achieve tension and/or relaxation should be covered. Therapists assign home practice only after adequate discussion of this first practice experience.

## Initial Progressive Relaxation Home Practice

Therapists ask clients to conduct formal PRT practice sessions at home on a daily basis. Bernstein et al. (2000) recommended twice daily home practice sessions at least 3 hours apart. Many motivated clients eager to learn therapy techniques comply with this request. However, clients expressing concern about keeping up with anxiety self-monitoring and other home practice assignments might benefit from planning only one daily relaxation practice from the beginning. Assigning once daily practice for these clients may increase the likelihood that they follow through and honor their home practice commitment. Therapists can explain that twice daily practice is the best way to develop relaxation skills quickly and then ask clients if they are willing to make such a commitment. If clients raise concerns about complying with two daily home practice sessions, therapists can work with them to make sure one daily practice is scheduled. These clients also can experiment with adding a second practice session after they have established a once-daily practice routine.

Initial home practice sessions follow the same format as the therapist-guided practice session. Clients typically conduct their first few home practice sessions listening to the initial PRT practice session audiotape on a stereo or with headphones. Practice with the audiotape helps clients learn the sequence of muscle groups, instructions for producing tension in each, and the timing of tension-release cycles. However, therapists must instruct clients to stop use of the tape as soon as the practice sequence is learned. Clients need the experience of creating tension and relaxation on their own to master muscle relaxation skills. Clients should be warned against becoming dependent on the tape to achieve states of deep relaxation. For this reason, clients should practice without the audiotape by the third or fourth day of practice. Clients continue daily home practice of the 16 muscle group procedure without the audiotape until they easily achieve deep relaxation in all muscle groups on a consistent basis. Such skill mastery typically takes two to three weeks of regular and frequent formal home practice.

The following instructions are reviewed with clients before they begin formal home PRT practice:

1. Conduct each practice in a quiet and comfortable place where you will not be disturbed. Select a comfortable chair, such as a padded recliner chair, or a bed. Make any necessary arrangements ahead of time, such as asking others in your home not to disturb you, turning off the telephone ringer and television, or making a trip to the bathroom.
2. Loosen any tight clothing and remove your watch, jewelry, shoes, eyeglasses, and anything else that creates pressure on your body.
3. Begin each practice session by giving yourself a few seconds to settle down after closing your eyes. When you are ready, start the audiotape and follow the muscle tension and release instructions carefully. Be sure to stop using the audiotape as soon as you have learned the procedure and can guide yourself through from memory.
4. Direct all your attention to the current muscle group and the physical sensations of tension and relaxation you create. As you notice your mind wandering from the present moment, gently bring it back to the sensations of tension or relaxation in the current muscle group.
5. When you relax each muscle group, be sure to release all tension immediately rather than gradually.
6. Try not to move a muscle group after you have finished relaxation for that group. Go ahead and move whenever you need to feel comfortable, but avoid any unnecessary movements and remain as still as possible during the practice session.
7. Rate your anxiety just before and immediately after each home practice session.
8. Schedule practice sessions during waking hours rather than just before falling asleep at night. Effective relaxation skill development requires learning how to relax your muscles in a wakeful state. Eventually you will practice applying this relaxation skill while awake in daily life.

### Subsequent Progressive Relaxation Training Procedures

Once clients have mastered the initial 16 muscle group procedure, therapists demonstrate how to combine muscle groups down to 7 muscle groups. The 7 muscle groups recommended by Bernstein et al. (2000) are as follows:

1. Right (dominant) hand and forearm are combined with the right upper arm.
2. Left (nondominant) hand and forearm are combined with the left upper arm.
3. The three facial muscle groups are combined together.
4. The neck and throat remain a separate muscle group.
5. The chest, shoulders, and back are combined with the abdomen.
6. Right (dominant) upper leg, calf, and foot are combined together.
7. Left (nondominant) upper leg, calf, and foot are combined together.

If time allows, therapists can guide clients through formal practice of this 7 muscle group procedure in session. As before, if therapists decide to audiotape this new procedure, clients should discontinue use of the tape at home as soon as they learn the new sequence. Clients continue their daily home practice sessions following the same instructions as before but replace the full 16 muscle group procedure with the new 7 muscle group procedure.

After clients have mastered this abbreviated practice, typically after two or three weeks of frequent and regular practice, therapists introduce a further abbreviated 4 muscle group procedure. The 4 muscle group PRT version by Bernstein et al. (2000) is as follows:

1. The right and left hands, forearms, and upper arms are combined.
2. The facial muscles are combined with the neck.
3. The muscles of the chest, shoulders, back, and abdomen remain a separate group.
4. The right and left upper legs, calves, and feet are combined.

Therapists again can guide clients through in-session practice of this procedure if time allows. Audiotape is usually not necessary, as most clients can remember the 4 muscle group sequence after this first formal practice session. Clients should practice this new 4 muscle group relaxation procedure at home daily until they are able to produce the same degree of relaxation experienced during the original 16 muscle group procedure.

Following mastery of the 4 muscle group practice, clients advance to relaxation recall procedures. Rather than producing tension during formal practice, clients systematically focus attention on each of the 4 muscle groups to identify any feelings of residual tension. Once tension has been detected, clients recall what complete relaxation felt like in those muscles as they release all tension immediately. Therapists typically guide clients through this procedure in session, reviewing each of the 4 muscle groups as clients scan these muscles for any tightness, recall feelings of relaxation, and produce relaxation by releasing all tension. Clients then practice this recall procedure at home for at least one week.

After clients achieve deep relaxation from this new recall procedure, therapists add a counting procedure. Bernstein et al. (2000) recommended that clients end recall practice sessions by covertly counting from one to ten slowly. With each count, clients become more and more deeply relaxed. Therapists can guide clients through this procedure in session before assigning home practice of recall with counting. Eventually clients practice relaxation by simply counting from one to ten. During this count, clients systematically focus attention on each muscle group while allowing the muscles throughout the body to relax more deeply with each count. With practice, many clients learn to achieve deep muscle relaxation by counting alone. This final procedure teaches clients a method for achieving muscle relaxation quickly. Thus, clients can make use of their progressive relaxation skills throughout the day to reduce baseline levels of muscle tension. In addition, clients can apply muscle relaxation skills as a coping response to stressful situations and early anxiety spiral cues.

## *Alternative Progressive Relaxation Training Procedures*

Other variations of the original Jacobsonian PRT technique have been incorporated into GAD treatment protocols. For example, Barlow and colleagues begin with essentially the same 16 muscle groups as Bernstein et al. (2000) but arrange the muscle groups in a different order with some differences in tensing instructions (Craske & Barlow 2006a; Zinbarg, Craske, & Barlow 2006). Similar to the Bernstein et al. method, the 16 muscle groups are later reduced to eight. Eventually clients focus their relaxation practice on 4 muscle groups considered most relevant to GAD: the abdomen, chest, shoulders, and forehead. Clients then add a counting procedure, ultimately learning to achieve a state of relaxation within the count of five in response to situational cues.

In their GAD treatment protocol, Rygh and Sanderson (2004) presented a progressive muscle relaxation procedure first described by Klosko and Sanderson (1999). Clients begin with formal practice of tension-release cycles including 15 muscle groups. Clients later practice the 15 muscle group procedure without producing tension, only relaxing each muscle group systematically during formal practice. These 15 muscle groups resemble the 16 muscle groups of Bernstein et al. (2000), but some differences can be found. Muscles of the hips are included, the arrangement and sequence of muscle groups differ, and alternative tensing instructions for certain muscle groups are offered.

A final progressive relaxation training procedure described by Leahy and Holland (2000) begins with only 12 muscle groups. This method encompasses the same muscles as the Bernstein et al. (2000) 16 muscle group procedure. All muscles are combined down to eight for further practice. Clients then focus their practice efforts on 4 specific muscle groups consisting of the arms, upper chest and back, shoulders and neck, and the face. Eventually relaxation through recall and counting procedures are practiced so that clients can respond to reminder cues with relaxation over the course of the day.

Some clinicians find the full Bernstein et al. (2000) PRT procedure too extensive to administer when a limited number of treatment sessions are available. Indeed, some managed care settings do not allow even ten therapy sessions, the length of time recommended by Bernstein and colleagues for optimal relaxation skill development. However, with strategic planning, therapists could provide clients with essential information and relaxation training experiences using very little session time. Clients could read a therapist handout containing the PRT rationale before session to reduce the amount of session time needed to introduce the technique. After therapist demonstration of muscle tension instructions and the first in-session practice, clients could follow the subsequent steps on their own with simple therapist instructions. Many motivated clients might enjoy substantial benefits from regular and frequent home practice of the 16 muscle group, 7 muscle group, 4 muscle group, and relaxation by recall and counting procedures. When therapist contact is even more limited, clients can learn progressive relaxation on their own with self-help methods. A single progressive relaxation exercise condensing all Bernstein et al. (2000) 16 muscle groups down to five appears in

Hazlett-Stevens (2005), *Women who worry too much.* Likewise, the Client Workbook of *Mastery of your anxiety and worry, 2nd edition* (MAW-2; Craske & Barlow 2006a) contains specific instructions for home practice of their alternative progressive relaxation training method.

## Imagery Relaxation Training

This final relaxation technique is particularly relevant to GAD. Given the verbal-linguistic nature of worry, many of these clients do not engage in visual imagery often. Indeed, distressing images may be one type of internal experience worry serves to avoid (Borkovec, Alcaine, & Behar 2004). Teaching clients to relax through pleasant imagery increases the frequency of this specific cognitive activity in a non-threatening context. Imagery relaxation practice also prepares clients for the imagery exposure strategies presented later in treatment. Thus, the purpose of imagery relaxation training is twofold. First, this technique teaches clients a third way to achieve relaxation. This particular relaxation method develops a previously untapped internal resource, the innate human ability to visualize. Second, pleasant imagery acquaints clients with this previously avoided covert activity before more threatening images are introduced in treatment. Once clients learn to generate relaxing images, their newly developed imagery skills are applied in subsequent imaginal exposure exercises.

Imagery relaxation training can be introduced early in treatment and does not take long to teach. After a brief rationale, therapists help clients select a specific scene expected to create a subjective state of relaxation. Therapists then guide clients through visualization of this scene in session, encouraging clear and vivid imagery involving all of the senses. Following discussion of client experience and repeated practice, therapists assign relaxation imagery home practice.

### *Imagery Relaxation Rationale*

Therapists introduce imagery as a way to create deep feelings of relaxation using only the mind. Through mental imagery, clients can create a vivid visual picture that affects the body and mind in powerful ways. Visualization is likened to a natural form of virtual reality, whereas other types of thinking such as worry involve talking to the self in words. Imagery therefore elicits deeper states of relaxation as well as other emotions than verbal-linguistic thinking can. Imagery relaxation exercises teach clients to capitalize on this effect for the purpose of coping with anxiety spirals. In addition, imagery will provide a way to confront feared situations in later therapy sessions. Development of imagery skills will increase the likelihood that clients will benefit from this exposure therapy component as well.

Imagery relaxation training is very straightforward. Clients simply choose a scene they expect will be particularly relaxing for them and then practice visualizing this scene as vividly as possible for short periods of time. With repeated practice, the imagery becomes more and more vivid and clients require less and less time to achieve a state of deep relaxation. Formal practice of this final relaxation strategy will be incorporated into other relaxation home practice assignments. Eventually clients will have developed yet another way to relax themselves throughout the day or in response to anxiety cues and triggers.

## Imagery Relaxation Session Procedures

Therapists next ask clients to decide upon a relaxing scene. Clients should select a specific place containing explicit visual stimuli. However, the scene does not have to represent an actual place clients have visited. Any place outdoors with natural beauty can be used for imagery relaxation. Common examples include the beach, a green meadow or field of favorite flowers, a forest of pine trees, snow-covered mountains, or the sun rising or setting over a desert landscape. Therapists ask clients to describe their scene in great detail before imagery practice begins. For example, if the client selected a beach scene, where exactly on the beach are they sitting? What time of day is it and what are the weather conditions? What body of water are they viewing? Is the water calm or with active waves? What is the color of the water, the sand, and the sky? What other scenery can be seen, such as trees, rocks, or grass? Once clients can describe several visual details, therapists ask questions about other sensations that can be experienced during scene imagination. Tactile sensations, such as the texture of the sand or the temperature of a breeze in the air, should be discussed. Therapists and clients also should identify any sounds or smells that would accompany the scene.

After clients have described their scene in sufficient detail, therapists proceed with the formal practice of imagery relaxation. Therapists invite clients to get physically comfortable in the chair and to close their eyes. Therapists then instruct clients to turn on the relaxing image using a cue word that reminds clients of their selected scene. Therapists ask clients to picture themselves in the scene as vividly as possible, as if they were really there right now. During this imagery practice, therapists facilitate clear and vivid imagery by describing details of the scene generated earlier. The following sample therapy transcript demonstrates a therapist guiding a client through this portion of the first practice attempt.

> Therapist: Go ahead and close your eyes…get as comfortable as you can in the chair…and turn on your beach image now…picture yourself there on the beach… create as vivid an image as you can as if you're really there right now…as you gaze into the deep blue ocean…listening to the rhythm of the waves as they crash against the rocks…feeling the warmth of the sun on your skin just before a gentle breeze touches your face…smelling the salt water in the air as your breathe in… just sitting there on the beach with nothing to do but enjoy your surroundings…

After approximately 30 seconds, therapists instruct clients to turn off the image and remain still with their eyes closed as they continue to relax. After another 30 seconds, therapists request that clients open their eyes and describe their imagery. Therapists ask how well clients were able to create a vivid image and to experience the scene as if they were actually there. Clients reporting difficulty simply try again as therapists describe the scene in greater detail. Repeated practice in session continues until clients report that they created a vivid image immediately and were able to stay in the scene until instructed to stop visualizing the image. Clients exhibiting poor imagery ability at first often respond to therapist encouragement and repeated practice attempts. Therapists can reassure these clients by explaining that little of their usual mental activity involves imagery, so imagery exercises can feel unfamiliar and difficult at first. However, imagery is just another new skill that will develop with practice.

## *Imagery Relaxation Home Practice*

Clients can add formal home practice of imagery relaxation training to other relaxation home practice. For example, clients can switch from the present-moment focus task to imagery practice at the end of their 10-min diaphragmatic breathing home practice sessions. Clients also could imagine their relaxing scene at the end of progressive relaxation home practice. When the time to practice imagery arrives, clients turn on the image immediately as they say a cue word to themselves representing the scene (e.g., "beach," "mountains"). Just as they practiced in session, clients create as vivid an image as possible and stay in the scene for approximately 30 seconds. Clients imagine as many sights, sounds, smells, and tactile sensations as they can during scene imagination. Eventually clients develop strong imagery skills which produce deep relaxation within a brief imagery period.

## Combining Relaxation Techniques

Clients learn all three relaxation strategies so they have multiple relaxation response options at any moment. They later experiment with all three, discovering for themselves which technique(s) work best in certain situations or in response to certain cues. However, each relaxation skill requires dedicated effort and repeated practice before becoming effective. Clients quickly become overwhelmed when multiple relaxation home practice assignments are added to ongoing self-monitoring and other therapy assignments. For this reason, the three relaxation strategies are presented one at a time in separate therapy sessions. Home practice assignments are combined into one formal home practice procedure, allowing clients to practice more than one skill without having to schedule several formal practice sessions per day.

As early as the first treatment session, therapists teach diaphragmatic breathing as described above. Clients practice only this relaxation technique at home twice per day over the next one to two weeks. Meanwhile, therapy continues with psychoeducation, review of self-monitoring, and initial cognitive therapy proce-dures. As clients gain mastery over this first relaxation skill and incorporate dia-phragmatic breathing into their daily life, therapists proceed with progressive relaxation and assign formal home practice of the 16 muscle group procedure. Clients continue formal diaphragmatic breathing practice by adding this proce-dure to the end of their progressive relaxation home practice sessions. Once cli-ents have mastered 16 muscle group progressive relaxation procedures, therapists introduce imagery relaxation training in session. Imagery home practice is then added to the end of each formal home practice, immediately following progres-sive relaxation and diaphragmatic breathing procedures. Home practice of subse-quent progressive muscle relaxation procedures (i.e., 7 muscle group, 4 muscle group, recall, and counting procedures) also are followed by diaphragmatic breathing and imagery relaxation practice. As clients master these relaxation skills, they practice applying each in daily life. Clients periodically return to formal home practice sessions to enhance skill development and to maintain relaxation skills over time.

## Applying Relaxation Techniques

Therapists assign formal home practice sessions so that clients develop strong relaxation skills. These skills become useful when incorporated into daily life. In the treatment of GAD, the ultimate aim for each relaxation technique is its deployment in response to anxiety cues and stressful situations. This application of relaxation training dates back to systematic desensitization, the behavior therapy for phobias developed by Wolpe (1958). Clients learned progressive relaxation so they could produce a relaxation response quickly when confronting specific anxiety-provoking stimuli in later exposure treatment sessions. Öst (1987) expanded this progressive relaxation application to a variety of naturally occurring anxiety-provoking situa-tions. His applied relaxation therapy procedures have received empirical support for the treatment of several phobias, panic disorder, chronic pain, and other medical conditions (see Öst 1987 and Bernstein et al. 2000 for reviews of this literature). Empirical support also exists for applied relaxation as a treatment for GAD (e.g., Öst & Breitholtz 2000; Arntz 2003). However, applied relaxation appears most effective for GAD as a component of a larger cognitive-behavioral treatment package (Borkovec & Ruscio 2001; Gould, Safren, Washington, & Otto 2004). Not surprisingly, variations of the Öst (1987) applied relaxation technique are found in most cognitive-behavioral GAD treatment package protocols (Zinbarg, Craske, & Barlow 2006 and Craske & Barlow 2006a; Rygh & Sanderson 2004; Leahy & Holland 2000). The version described below is based on the procedures developed by Borkovec and colleagues (Borkovec, Newman, Pincus, & Lytle 2002; Bernstein et al. 2000).

Clients learn to apply their relaxation skills in three specific ways. First, when clients detect increases in anxiety or subtle anxiety cues during self-monitoring, they immediately respond with relaxation strategies including present-moment focus of attention. Second, clients relax many times per day in response to everyday reminder cues. Finally, clients practice relaxation during short breaks scheduled ahead of time. All three applications help clients remain as relaxed as feasible throughout the day. Eventually clients incorporate newly acquired relaxation skills into their lifestyle on a permanent basis. Therapists introduce these applied relaxation procedures after clients have developed adequate relaxation skills through formal home practice assignments.

## Relaxation Coping Responses

This primary relaxation training application integrates relaxation responses into the anxiety self-monitoring procedures described in the previous chapter. Relaxation becomes a coping response whenever clients detect early anxiety cues during the course of regular anxiety self-monitoring. Therapists instruct clients to practice relaxing in the moment each time their anxiety rating reveals a shift away from a relaxed state. Each time clients record an anxiety rating, they bring their attention back to the present moment and current bodily sensations. Clients immediately shift to slow diaphragmatic breathing and scan the 4 muscle groups for any excess tension to relax away. If circumstances allow, clients also might retreat for 30–60 seconds to close their eyes and engage in pleasant imagery. Imagery relaxation requires clients' full attention and therefore cannot be used while performing divided attention tasks such as driving or talking to others. For this reason, this relaxation technique cannot be deployed in the midst of a stressful situation demanding client attention and behavioral responses. However, if clients can afford the brief time needed for pleasant imagery, the resulting quick return to a relaxed state might help them orient to the problem or task at hand effectively.

Therapists model this relaxation application for clients during therapy sessions, just as they modeled frequent anxiety monitoring in previous sessions. Each time an anxiety rating is reported, therapists ask clients to spend the next few moments bringing their mind back to the present. During this time, clients focus on their breathing, shift to diaphragmatic breathing, and scan their muscles, letting go of any excess muscle tension. Clients also might close their eyes and imagine their relaxing scene.

Therapists and clients explore any upcoming situations or possible scenarios in which brief relaxation coping responses would be helpful. Identifying such situations ahead of time increases the likelihood that clients will remember to attempt a relaxation response when the time arrives. For example, a client concerned about an upcoming work meeting might plan to practice diaphragmatic breathing and muscle relaxation briefly at her desk just before walking to the meeting room. During the meeting, she could shift back to diaphragmatic breathing each time another person is talking.

## *Relaxation Reminder Cues*

In addition to scheduled written anxiety ratings, clients are encouraged to self-monitor anxiety at other times throughout the day. Clients conduct this informal self-monitoring using external reminder cues such as every hour on the hour, each time the phone rings, or each time a different task begins at work. Other examples include watching a commercial on television or walking from a parked car. Instances in which clients find themselves waiting for a few moments also can serve as reminders to self-monitor. Possibilities include waiting in line, sitting at a red light while driving, waiting for a computer to boot up, waiting for a pot of water to boil, or waiting in the car when picking kids up from school. These external cues first used as reminders to self-monitor now become reminders to relax as well. Clients immediately deploy diaphragmatic breathing and progressive relaxation strategies, and if appropriate, pleasant imagery each time these events occur. Therapists should review likely external reminder cues with clients and ask them to select a few specific cues common to their daily activities. From now on, each time clients encounter a situational cue, they remind themselves to rate their anxiety and to relax.

Clients also monitor themselves for any internal cues or behaviors that signal a need to relax. As clients notice worry or muscle tension, these symptoms can remind them to practice an immediate relaxation response. Each time clients find themselves fidgeting, biting their fingernails, skin picking, playing with their hair, sighing heavily, cracking their knuckles, talking quickly, or tapping their feet, their own behavior serves as a reminder to relax. Each week therapists encourage clients to discover earlier and earlier cues that can serve this new purpose. Old anxiety habits therefore take on the new function of reminding clients to implement relaxation coping responses. Each time clients notice cognitive, somatic, or behavioral anxiety cues they can practice slow and deep stomach breathing and release any unnecessary muscle tension. Therapists can model this relaxation application during therapy sessions as well. Whenever therapists note client verbal or nonverbal anxiety cues, facial muscle tension, or anxious behavior, they can mention this observation, ask about current anxiety spiral components, and invite clients to practice brief relaxation.

## *Daily Brief Relaxation Practice*

Frequent brief practice sessions help clients maintain baseline states of relaxation throughout the day. Clients respond to everyday demands and challenging situations more effectively while relaxed. In addition, the simple act of purposefully taking a break from routine activities provides a respite from anxious experience and the hassles of everyday life. Indeed, many clients report enjoyment of formal home practice sessions at first for this reason.

Therapists and clients discuss a typical daily routine and identify when clients might schedule short breaks lasting 3–5 min each throughout the day. During these breaks, clients retreat to any available quiet place and practice present-moment focus of attention, diaphragmatic breathing, and progressive relaxation. Imagery relaxation also can be practiced during these scheduled mini breaks. Clients working away from home during the day might locate an outdoor courtyard or an empty lounge area where they can retreat for these short breaks. Other clients might choose a favorite room at home, a garden, or a park bench for brief relaxation practice. During each mini break, clients devote all their attention to their relaxation practice. Clients practice either present-moment focus on sensations of breathing and muscle relaxation or pleasant imagery. These breaks should be spaced throughout the daytime hours as much as possible, such as mid-morning, lunchtime, mid-afternoon, and early evening. If clients prefer, these mini breaks can coincide with written anxiety self-monitoring entries.

## Chapter Summary

Relaxation training targets the somatic component of anxiety spirals, teaching clients a coping response to anxiety cues and a means for reducing baseline levels of tension. These strategies might be conceptualized as essential emotion regulation skills many clients suffering from GAD did not develop naturally. Relaxation practice requires clients to focus attention on the present moment, complementing mindfulness therapy approaches. This specific aspect of relaxation training seems especially pertinent to GAD, given the future-oriented nature of worry. Therefore, explicit instructions to re-focus the mind on present moment sensations or mental tasks such as counting have been incorporated into relaxation training procedures.

The relaxation strategies most widely used and studied in GAD treatment include diaphragmatic breathing, progressive (muscle) relaxation, and pleasant imagery. Therapists teach each strategy beginning with a brief rationale and in-session demonstration of the technique. Clients then complete daily formal home practice assignments in a quiet, undisturbed setting to build relaxation skills. As relaxation skills develop from formal practice, clients learn to apply these skills in daily life. Diaphragmatic breathing teaches clients the difference between fast, shallow chest breathing and slow, deep stomach breathing. Chest breathing is associated with subtle hyperventilation and anxiety-like physiology, whereas abdominal breathing promotes feelings of relaxation. Formal home practice sessions include a present-moment focus task. Later applications of this relaxation technique involve an immediate shift to diaphragmatic breathing in response to increased anxiety, internal anxiety cues, or external reminder cues. Progressive relaxation training begins with systematic tension and release of 16 specific muscle groups. As clients gain experience with this full procedure, muscles are combined down to seven, and eventually four, larger groups. Clients later practice relaxation through recall by scanning each muscle group and releasing without first producing tension. Counting procedures are added so clients learn to achieve deep muscle relaxation quickly. Relaxation imagery teaches clients to generate a clear and vivid image. Clients select a relaxing scene and practice immersing themselves in associated sights, sounds, smells, and tactile sensations for approximately 30 seconds. Applied relaxation integrates relaxation training into anxiety self-monitoring. Clients quickly relax as a coping response to anxiety cues and stressful situations. Therapists also help clients identify everyday external cues that can serve as reminders to relax. Finally, clients incorporate each relaxation strategy into daily life by scheduling short breaks throughout the day for brief practice.

# Chapter 6
# Cognitive Strategies

Systematic methods for challenging and restructuring dysfunctional cognition first appeared in the 1950's and 1960's. Albert Ellis developed one of the first such therapies, Rational Emotive Behavior Therapy (REBT; Ellis 1962), as he observed the complex interaction between thoughts, feelings, and behavior. REBT teaches clients they can choose to react to adversity with rational beliefs that promote adaptive behavior. Disputing rigid "irrational" beliefs therefore lies at the heart of this therapy approach. However, the cognitive component found in most anxiety disorder treatments stems from the cognitive therapy of Aaron T. Beck and colleagues (Beck, Rush, Shaw, & Emery 1979; Beck, Emery, & Greenberg 1985). According to this model, maladaptive emotional distress results from inflexible negative interpretations of various situations or stimuli. In particular, excessive anxiety is caused by repeatedly overestimating threat while underestimating coping resources. Cognitive therapy therefore teaches clients to examine surrounding evidence in an objective way. As faulty interpretations are addressed, this negative interpretation bias reduces and destructive attributions decrease.

Beck and colleagues (1979) proposed that feelings and behavior are mostly determined by ways in which individuals construe and perceive their world, self, and future (i.e., "cognitive triad"). Although fundamental belief systems developed from previous experiences, destructive "schemas" generate problematic cognition in response to present-day events. As individuals interpret current experience negatively, emotional distress and behavior consistent with their negative appraisals result. A self-fulfilling prophecy is therefore created: negative perceptions are strengthened by negative feelings and maladaptive behavioral consequences. Core beliefs about personal incompetence and inadequacy are commonly found among depressed individuals. Interestingly, this same theme distinguished the worry of individuals endorsing GAD diagnostic criteria from nonanxious individuals (Hazlett-Stevens & Craske 2003b). Thus, a view of the self as incompetent integrated with views of the world and the future as threatening are the primary cognitive characteristics of GAD.

Cognitive therapy is based on the premise that thoughts are simply products of the mind which may or may not validly reflect external reality. The popular cognitive therapy adage "a thought is just a thought" conveys this view of cognition as subjective perception rather than fact. As clients become aware of automatic anxious

H. Hazlett-Stevens, *Psychological Approaches to Generalized Anxiety Disorder*, doi: 10.1007/978-0-387-76870-0, © Springer Science + Business Medic, LLC 2008

thoughts through daily thought tracking, they appreciate the subjective nature of their cognition. This new approach contrasts with old habits of reacting to each thought as if it represented factual reality. Thus, one purpose of cognitive therapy is cognitive distancing, or teaching clients to view their thoughts as mere guesses, hypotheses, and predictions. This initial step reveals the complexity and ambiguity inherent in many real-life situations clients often overlook. Beck et al. (1979) described depressed cognition as invariant, containing absolute and nondimensional judgments. Similarly, GAD has been linked to a lack of cognitive flexibility (Hazlett-Stevens 1997, 2000), and both state and trait worry disrupted ambiguous task performance (Metzger, Miller, Cohen, Sofka, & Borkovec 1990). Furthermore, Dugas and colleagues identified intolerance of uncertainty as a causal risk factor for GAD (see Dugas & Robichaud 2007 for a review). While cognitive therapy reduces threat perceptions by challenging specific anxious thoughts, this treatment component also may address underlying fears of ambiguity and uncertainty specific to GAD.

In GAD treatment, cognitive therapy targets elevated perceptions of threat. The cognitive component of anxiety spirals are identified and challenged, allowing for more balanced perspectives. As anxious thoughts occur, clients learn they can choose subsequent reactions. Thoughts are examined objectively so that adaptive behavior can be selected over reflexive responses. Clients also become aware of any underlying assumptions and beliefs driving excessive worry and other anxious behavior. For example, views of the self as incompetent are restructured. Beliefs about the need to worry are discussed and tested. Eventually clients adopt more flexible and adaptive cognitive styles that replace excessive worry and hypervigilance.

Given the uncertain and subjective nature of cognition, Beck and colleagues (1979) recommended a therapy process termed "collaborative empiricism." That is, the cognitive therapist encourages active client participation in the construction of empirical investigations. Automatic thoughts, interpretations of events, and underlying beliefs are tested objectively instead of accepted blindly. Clients and therapists work together to identify hidden appraisals or assumptions then examine each in a scientific fashion. During sessions, therapists challenge automatic thoughts with Socratic questions revealing critical information or alternative perspectives clients had not considered. Specific therapy techniques teach clients adaptive ways of examining their automatic anxious thoughts. Home assignments encourage practice of these new responses and sometimes involve gathering additional evidence before making judgments and final conclusions. Cognitive therapists create a trusting therapeutic relationship with warmth and empathy, interacting with clients in a genuine way. Beck and colleagues famously claimed that such therapist characteristics are "necessary but not sufficient" for therapy success.

Cognitive therapy procedures begin early in treatment and typically continue until therapy termination. As early as the second therapy session, therapists introduce the cognitive therapy rationale and help clients identify specific anxious thoughts. Clients practice this initial step between sessions with thought tracking procedures. Each time clients detect an anxious thought or worry, they either solve a concrete problem by taking constructive action or they postpone the worry to a designated "worry period." In later sessions, therapists challenge anxious thoughts with specific cognitive techniques. During this process, therapists and clients discover overarching worry themes, underlying assumptions, and core beliefs. Beliefs about worry itself are examined as well. This cognitive material is challenged and tested using the same procedures as before. Finally, clients learn to generate alternative, more balanced, perspectives. The procedures described in this chapter teach clients a systematic method for examining and challenging their anxious thoughts. Cognitive strategies become another portable coping skill clients can apply whenever they encounter stressful situations or detect anxiety cues in daily life.

## Initial Cognitive Therapy Procedures

Like most CBT components, therapists introduce cognitive therapy to clients with a brief rationale. Once clients understand its nature and purpose, therapists present a method for tracking anxious thoughts between sessions. The first step to successful cognitive therapy is identification of specific anxious thoughts. Therapists teach clients to narrow each worry down to a concrete interpretation or prediction. Such specificity allows for subsequent empirical examination. In addition, clients practice a new response to initial worry detection. As self-monitoring and thought tracking reveal in-the-moment anxious thoughts, clients determine whether concrete problem-solving can occur. If so, they shift to constructive action in that moment. If not, the worry is recorded and postponed to a scheduled worry period later that day. Clients then redirect their attention back to the present moment and resume whatever activity they were engaged in when the worry began.

### *Cognitive Therapy Rationale*

Therapists present cognitive therapy as a way to target anxious thoughts and worry directly. Just as relaxation strategies target the physiological component of anxiety spirals, cognitive therapy targets the cognitive component by putting worries and anxious thoughts in perspective. Therapists explain the basic tenet of cognitive therapy: Our thoughts are interpretations of events or predictions about the future that directly impact how we feel. Therapists provide examples of ambiguous situations that could be perceived in multiple ways and therefore lead to different emotions. In one popular hypothetical example, a man unexpectedly sees a neighbor while shopping out in public. Although the neighbor indeed saw the man, she did not say "hello" or otherwise acknowledge him. Importantly, the way the man interpreted this interaction determined how he felt. If he assumed the neighbor was preoccupied with her own problems, he would feel sympathy and compassion. If he believed the neighbor was ignoring him because she thought she was "better" than him, he would feel angry. If he thought his neighbor was upset with him because he must have said something offensive, he might feel anxious or guilty. Clients are invited to think of examples from their own experience. When discussing each example, therapists emphasize how a particular interpretation led to a certain feeling and behavioral response. However, there were several different possible interpretations for each situation.

In the case of GAD, ambiguous situations are often interpreted as threatening. Much research has shown that people who struggle with anxiety and worry are prone to see danger when faced with ambiguous stimuli or events (see MacLeod & Rutherford 2004 for a review). When this happens, feelings of anxiety and apprehension result. Clients feel as if the threat were real even though their feelings are based only on an illusion of danger. Clients are then encouraged to think of a recent experience when they interpreted an ambiguous situation in an anxiety-provoking way only to find there was no actual threat. Therapists emphasize that clients felt the same emotions as they would had their interpretation been accurate. Because they are biased toward threatening interpretations, they are more likely to respond to ambiguity with anxiety. Furthermore, everyone is more likely to interpret ambiguous things as threatening when they're already anxious. Anxious feelings and anxious thoughts therefore work together in a reciprocal feedback loop, each one increasing the chances of the other.

Many situations in everyday life are filled with ambiguity. Social interactions, one of the main types of situations people worry about, contain numerous verbal and non-verbal cues that can be interpreted in multiple ways. The future is always uncertain to some degree due to the simple fact it has not yet happened. Not surprisingly, these high-ambiguity realms are most problematic for people prone to threatening interpretations. Eventually uncertainty in and of itself becomes feared as ambiguity becomes equated with threat. Worry might even become a way to cope with uncertainty, making the future seem more certain, but therefore more dangerous, than it truly might be. Beliefs that clients need to worry to prepare for the worst or to prevent future disaster develop. Cognitive therapy teaches clients to explore many possible perspectives, increasing acceptance of life's uncertainties. Clients let go of their worries as they discover they don't really need worry to cope with uncertain events and outcomes.

An important property of anxiety-provoking thoughts is that they happen very quickly and are often barely noticeable. These interpretations of threat have been rehearsed so many times, they become automatic. Like other anxiety spiral components, anxious thoughts are habits from the past. For this reason, clients may not even be aware of these thoughts when they occur. Nevertheless, clients respond with anxiety as if the automatic thought was valid and the threat is certain to happen. Worries are usually predictions about something bad happening in the future or negative interpretations of past events. The first goal of cognitive therapy is to identify exactly what clients' automatic thoughts are. This allows them to look at these thoughts objectively and to put them into perspective. Clients will learn that their anxious thoughts are only interpretations and predictions, not facts. They can view the future in a less anxiety-provoking way and discover they can cope with adversity even if it does happen.

After clients have learned to identify and examine automatic anxious thoughts, therapists help clients explore any underlying beliefs about themselves, the world, and the future that fuel anxious thoughts. Worry themes, rules or assumptions about themselves or others, and even beliefs about worry itself are identified and evaluated.

Basic views of the world as dangerous and of the self as unable to cope are common. Exaggerated fears of failure and believing that one is worthless or "not good enough" are other common examples. Many people who suffer from GAD have developed beliefs that harm would become more likely if they suddenly stopped worrying. All of these beliefs can be examined rather than accepted without question. Clients eventually generate more balanced perspectives and preventive beliefs.

## Identify Specific Anxious Thoughts

For cognitive therapy to be effective, clients first must identify the content of automatic anxious thoughts. Many clients initially struggle with this step because these thoughts happen very quickly outside of their awareness. Clients often experience worry as vague and abstract, oblivious to the discrete interpretations and predictions made. Yet when these specific cognitions occur out of awareness, they are believed wholeheartedly and acted upon. Each time clients notice worry and other anxiety spiral cues, they try to determine exactly what they are saying to themselves about the situation. How are they explaining the event to themselves such that they feel anxious? If worried about something in the future, exactly what do they fear will happen? Often clients worry about the future implications of a past event. In these cases, what specific repercussions are clients predicting for the future? Clients should continue their inquiry until they reach a concrete prediction or interpretation that is so specific an outside observer could factually conclude whether or not it occurred. Clients are warned against feeling discouraged at first and giving up. Although identifying specific thoughts sounds straightforward, this first step can be very difficult and take repeated practice.

Therapists help clients identify automatic thoughts in session before clients practice at home. One method involves asking clients to close their eyes and imagine a particular recent anxiety-provoking situation. Once clients have had a minute to immerse themselves in this image, therapists ask them to say aloud whatever thoughts and images pass through the mind. Questions such as "What do you envision happening?" or "What exactly would happen next?" might reveal futuristic predictions. Client descriptions of anxious interpretations are often subjective and intangible in nature. Statements such as "I looked like an idiot" can be followed up with therapist questions such as "What exactly did you do that you think made you look like an idiot?" or "What would another person see when you think you look like an idiot?" Clients who hesitate to respond are encouraged to take some educated guesses about what may have gone through their mind rather than search for the "right" answer. Therapists also might suggest some possible automatic thoughts and ask clients which seem most relevant. This process continues until clients articulate a concrete interpretation or prediction that can be subjected to empirical investigation.

Alternatively, therapists might construct a role play to elicit automatic thoughts. Therapists ask clients to pretend they are actually in a given situation while therapists respond in character. Clients say aloud what they fear happening next as well as what they are thinking to themselves as these thoughts occur. For example, a client worried about an upcoming work evaluation meeting with her supervisor might speak to the therapist as if the therapist were her supervisor in the meeting. Once clients put themselves directly into the situation through role play, automatic thoughts often become apparent to clients as well as to their therapists.

Beck and colleagues (1985) described a final method using a marker board. Clients give a few anxious thoughts in response to a main worry or fear. Therapists write each statement on the board verbatim, which typically triggers additional thoughts. As clients are given time to explore their anxious thoughts about the topic, more poignant and specific ones often follow. In addition, the experience of seeing such subjective cognitive activity written out in front of clients provides some initial distance from their thoughts.

If session time is too limited for the above procedures or if clients are exhibiting great difficulty in session, clients can attempt the following self-help exercise between sessions (Hazlett-Stevens 2005) reprinted in Fig. 6.1. This structured procedure helps clients narrow down an initial worry to a specific interpretation or prediction on their own. Clients write down their responses to each exercise step as they detect worry during their regular anxiety monitoring.

## Thought Tracking

Before automatic anxious thoughts are examined and challenged, clients practice catching these thoughts as they occur in the course of daily life. Thought tracking procedures provide a structured method for clients to identify and then to record specific anxious thoughts between sessions. Thought tracking forms prompt clients through subsequent steps as clients learn ways to challenge these automatic thoughts in later therapy sessions. Clients carry a thought tracking form with their anxiety monitoring form so that anxious thoughts can be recorded whenever detected. Each time clients notice they are worrying or feeling anxious, they take a moment to reflect on their cognitive activity. Just as they learned in session, clients try to identify a specific interpretation or prediction associated with that worry. What exactly are they are saying to themselves about the situation? How are they explaining the event to themselves such that they feel anxious? If worried about something in the future, exactly what do they fear will happen? Clients record as specific a statement as possible representing their anxious thought in the first column of their thought tracking form. The Thought Tracking Form developed at our University of Nevada, Reno chronic worry intervention program is provided in Client Handout 6.1.

Thought tracking compliments the anxiety self-monitoring clients started at the beginning of treatment. As clients become better at detecting anxiety spiral cues and situational triggers through regular monitoring, they become better able to respond to cues with this first cognitive therapy step. Once clients have identified a concrete interpretation or prediction, they have enabled themselves to see their anxious thought as only a guess or hypothesis rather than a fact. As they record each specific anxious thought, clients remind themselves to treat this specific thought as a guess, not a fact. The body and mind might react to the thought with anxiety very quickly, as if this

1. Pick a worry you've discovered today during your daily monitoring. Write this worry topic at the top of a new page in your journal. If you haven't yet started your regular daily monitoring, see the exercises in chapter 3 for specific instructions.
2. Underneath this general worry topic, write down a specific instance, event, or situation that best represents your recent worry. Get as detailed as you can.
3. Figure out if this worry is about the past or the future. Write down the following information:

   • Past event: If you're worrying about a situation that has already happened, how are you interpreting it or explaining it to yourself? What are you telling yourself about it that leaves you feeling anxious?
   • Future event: If your worry is about an upcoming situation or about something that could happen in the future, figure out exactly what you're predicting will happen or exactly what you fear could happen. This should be so specific that another person could objectively see whether or not this event has occurred at a later point in time.

4. Now try to get your anxious thought as specific as you possibly can. Be on the lookout for these obstacles to getting specific:

   • General terms: Watch out for general terms that have subjective meaning to you but cannot be verified objectively. For example, if you're worried about a particular situation coming up in the future because you'll be a "failure," push yourself to clarify what you mean. What exactly are you predicting will happen when you use that word? Once that event has occurred, how will you be able to go back and determine whether or not the outcome you predicted has happened?
   • Unlimited time frame: Another trouble spot comes up when worries have a never-ending time frame. If this is the case for your current anxious thought, force yourself to find a point in the future that reflects when you think your prediction could happen or will have happened.

Once you have narrowed down what you are specifically worried about, summarize it in a sentence. Now make a column on the left side of the page, label it "Get Specific," and enter your sentence in this column under the Get Specific heading.

**Fig. 6.1** Identify Specific Anxious Thoughts Exercise. Reprinted with permission from New Harbinger Publications, Inc., and Holly Hazlett-Stevens, *Women Who Worry Too Much: How to Stop Worry and Anxiety from Ruining Relationships, Work, and Fun*, Hazlett-Stevens (2005)

thought were complete fact. This is why clients must make a conscious effort to remember that a thought is only a thought. It is just a guess or a hypothetical event created by the mind, even if it feels certain. Clients then decide to take constructive problem-solving action or to postpone their worry to an arranged time.

After clients record their specific anxious thought and remind themselves it is only a thought and not a fact, they determine whether constructive problem-solving can occur. Worry stems from the productive ability to think ahead, plan accordingly, and take constructive action. When people worry about a solvable concrete problem, they immediately can shift into problem solving about the situation in front of them. In this case, worry leads to action that provides a solution to a specific problem at hand. Each time an anxious thought is recorded, clients ask themselves if anything specific can be done to resolve the situation. For example, if the client just received a cancellation phone call from the babysitter but has plans to meet a friend for dinner, a problem has just presented itself to be solved. Rather than worrying unproductively and feeling increasingly anxious, the client can generate possible courses of action, weigh the

CLIENT HANDOUT 6.1. Thought tracking form

| Date | Step 1 | Step 2 | Step 3 | Step 4 | Step 5 | Step 6 |
|---|---|---|---|---|---|---|
| | Identify the specific anxious thought* | List alternative interpretations or predictions | Examine the likelihood and evidence | Decatastrophizing | Identify and examine core beliefs and worry beliefs | New perspectives and preventive beliefs |
| | | | | | | |
| | | | | | | |
| | | | | | | |
| | | | | | | |
| | | | | | | |
| | | | | | | |
| | | | | | | |

* **After you identify a specific anxious thought, immediately follow these steps:**
1. Remind yourself this is only a thought and not a fact.
2. Determine whether a concrete problem can be solved. If so, take constructive action to resolve the situation.
3. Otherwise, postpone your worry to your worry period. During your worry period, work through the remaining steps.

costs and benefits of each, and select the most desirable solution. The client might decide to call each babysitter on her back-up list to find a replacement, call her friend and reschedule the dinner, or ask her sister to come over and stay with her child. Whenever clients discover a specific problem under their control that can be solved, they can orient themselves to the problem and take subsequent action.

Individuals suffering from GAD tend to struggle with problem solving due to poor confidence in their ability to solve problems rather than problem-solving skill deficits (Ladouceur, Blais, Freeston, & Dugas 1998). Therefore, a tendency to react to concrete problems with self-doubt, worry, anxiety, and avoidance rather than constructive action sometimes occurs. Throughout cognitive therapy, clients are encouraged to act whenever they identify a concrete problem to solve. Each time an anxious thought is recorded on the Thought Tracking Form, clients determine whether or not they are worrying about a solvable problem at hand. This practice helps clients orient to the problem and perform constructive problem-solving behavior whenever useful.

## *Worry Postponement*

Most often, however, excessive worry represents vague concerns about the distant future, events outside an individual's control, or otherwise unsolvable problems. As discussed above, worry about uncontrollable uncertain events may develop as a strategy to cope with perceived threat and ambiguity. Davey (1994) described maladaptive worry as thwarted problem-solving. Unlike constructive worry, in which individuals anticipate specific problems and respond with task-oriented activity, "pathological" worry generates intrusive thoughts and excessive anxiety instead of adaptive behavior. For this reason, clients are instructed to re-direct their attention back to the present moment and delay the worry until their scheduled worry time arrives.

The clinical practice of postponing worry to a scheduled worry time originated as a stimulus control method (Borkovec, Wilkinson, Folensbee, & Lerman 1983). That is, limiting the worry process to a designated place and time could weaken its associations with various other external and internal stimuli. Given the pervasiveness of worry, this technique prevents worry responses from generalizing or spreading to new situations and stimuli. Thus, worry is contained to a specific set of situational cues selected ahead of time. Worry postponement also could be considered a response prevention technique (Rygh & Sanderson 2004) because clients are instructed to disengage from this cognitive activity whenever noticed. When successful, postponing a worry stops the anxiety spiral from developing further. Worry is viewed as a covert behavioral response over which clients gain control. As clients practice delaying worry to a worry period, they learn to disengage as well as to engage in worry as they choose. Finally, worry postponement might be conceptualized as applied mindfulness practice. Once detected, worries about the future serve as internal cues to bring the mind back to the present moment. Clients let go of their anxious thoughts and suspend any judgments about the situation until the scheduled worry period.

Client instructions for worry postponement are quite straightforward. When clients identify and record an anxious thought and determine there is no immediate concrete problem to be solved, they postpone the worry to a required "worry period." As clients detect worry throughout the day, they now have an alternative to getting caught up with worries as those worries appear. Instead, clients simply remind themselves they will revisit the worry during the worry period near the end of the day. Each time a worry is postponed, clients refocus their attention back to their immediate surroundings and the task at hand, experiencing the present moment as fully as possible. Clients schedule a 30-min worry period in the same place everyday. At the same time each day, clients retreat to their selected worry period location and review their worries of the day. Most clients select a comfortable place at home for the worry period, but any place incorporated into the client's routine might be possible. For example, clients might choose to conduct their worry period in an office at the end of the work day or while riding home on a commuter train. Clients should select a location where they can conduct their worry period on most days and can focus their attention on cognitive therapy practice without much distraction. At first, clients can spend this time simply thinking about their worries as they normally would. Soon clients will examine their anxious thoughts objectively and put them in perspective during the worry period. Clients will learn specific steps for challenging anxious thoughts in later sessions. Eventually clients will systematically work through each subsequent column on the Thought Tracking Form during their worry periods.

The worry postponement technique establishes a designated time for clients to complete cognitive therapy home assignments. Paradoxically, clients often find that the simple act of postponing a worry will render it insignificant by the time the worry period arrives. Sometimes the issue at hand becomes moot as circumstances change over the course of the day. Clients gain a sense of mastery over their worry, feeling they can choose when to address a worry and therefore do not need to eliminate worry altogether. For these reasons, the emotional intensity associated with spontaneous anxious thoughts tends to dissipate by the worry period. As one client explained, postponing her worry "took the wind right out of the sail." This practice fosters a greater acceptance of worries; clients discover they do not need to avoid or to fight each worry simply because it occurred. Worries can simply be postponed rather than engaged.

Therapists should caution clients against approaching worry postponement as a thought suppression strategy. Worry postponement is designed to teach clients a new response to their worry. Anxious thoughts are noticed, recorded, and then delayed to a later time. In contrast, suppressing anxious thoughts involves efforts to rid the mind of the thought immediately. Attempts at thought suppression, or purposefully trying not to think of something, often result in a paradoxical increase in unwanted thought frequency (see Wegner 1989 for a review). Below is a suggested therapist script from our University of Nevada, Reno chronic worry intervention program protocol designed to address this issue.

Therapist: It is important to realize that postponing worry is quite different from simply telling yourself to stop worrying. In fact, plenty of research shows that we are not very good at suppressing our thoughts, or purposefully trying NOT to think of something. Have you ever tried NOT to think of something? [Therapists discuss client responses to this question and each subsequent question in an interactive exchange.] For example, try NOT to think of a white bear. What happens if you try? In fact, the harder you try NOT to think of a white bear, the MORE you think of one, don't you? The same is true for worries…this is why "don't worry, be happy" doesn't work. Instead of trying to suppress anxious thoughts, just record each one when it occurs and promise yourself you'll come back to it during your worry period. If you think about it again, fine. If not, that's fine too. You'll have plenty of time to think about your worries later, knowing you'll come back to them during your worry period. Later on, you'll learn how to look at your worries objectively and put them in perspective during your worry period. For now, simply ask yourself if there is anything specific you can do to solve a concrete problem. If not, go ahead and postpone your worry. Once you have postponed your worry, make a concentrated effort to bring your mind back to the present moment. Try to focus all of your attention on whatever you were doing at the exact moment you caught yourself worrying.

## Specific Cognitive Techniques to Challenge Anxious Thoughts

Once clients are able to identify automatic anxious thoughts, these thoughts can be challenged. Various strategies question the validity and accuracy of client interpretations or predictions. However, cognitive therapy also exposes the many subtleties, ambiguities, and uncertainties inherent in everyday events. The ultimate aim of cognitive therapy for clients struggling with excessive worry is a greater appreciation for the rich complexity found in our world and ourselves. There are many ways to view a given situation, even an undesirable outcome. As clients experiment with multiple viewpoints, their cognitive flexibility increases. Eventually they learn to generate more balanced perspectives which incorporate subtle nuances of the situation. This goal significantly differs from mere thought substitution in which anxious thoughts are systematically replaced with positive thoughts.

Cognitive therapists select from an array of specific cognitive strategies as they challenge clients' anxious thoughts in session. Most of these strategies are applied with open-ended Socratic questioning. Therapists ask a series of pointed questions which expose information clients had not considered previously. Thus, therapists' questions encourage clients to expand narrow and fixed views. Therapists should not simply contradict or reject clients' anxious thoughts. Take the example of a client's specific anxious thought that she will be fired at her next job evaluation review. Rather than retorting that the client probably won't be fired, the therapist would ask questions such as "Why do you think you might be fired?" or "Is there any evidence to the contrary?" Therapists and clients then work together, either designing an empirical test of the initial anxious thought or otherwise examining it objectively. Over the course of several sessions, clients learn to ask such questions of themselves. Beck and colleagues (1985) characterized most automatic anxious thoughts as "Something bad is going to happen that I won't be able to handle." Cognitive therapists' subsequent questions are typically variants of three basic questions: (1) "What's the evidence?" (2) "What's another way of looking at the situation?" and (3) "So what if it happens?" (Beck et al. 1985, p. 201).

An advantage of this cognitive therapy process is the flexibility afforded to therapists. Any cognitive material therapists find fruitful can be pursued in the moment during the therapy session. However, a more structured approach to worry period assignments helps clients apply these techniques on their own. The Thought Tracking Form developed at our University of Nevada, Reno chronic worry intervention program systematically guides clients through a series of cognitive therapy steps. Therapists explain and demonstrate each step during therapy sessions. Clients self-apply each step during their subsequent worry periods between sessions. This method teaches cognitive strategies within a short period of time, making cognitive therapy accessible in managed care settings where therapy sessions might be limited. Clients first should experience some success with identifying automatic anxious thoughts, reminding themselves "thoughts are not facts," and postponing worry to a worry period if constructive problem-solving action was ruled out. Therapists then present specific cognitive techniques including: (1) generating alternative interpretations or predictions, (2) examining the likelihood and evidence, and (3) decatastrophizing. Clients systematically challenge each automatic anxious thought recorded on their Thought Tracking Forms during worry period practice.

## Generating Alternative Interpretations or Predictions

This technique maps onto Beck and colleagues' (1985) second question, "What's another way of looking at the situation?" Specific interpretations of past events and specific predictions about future events are all uncertain to some degree. Specific predictions reflecting future consequences of a past event are also unknown. Therefore, each automatic anxious thought represents only one of many possibilities. Therapists illustrate this point by encouraging clients to generate as many different interpretations or predictions as they can. In the spirit of true brainstorming, clients state each possibility as it occurs to them regardless of how outlandish, absurd, or unlikely the alternative may seem. Logical analysis and likelihood judgments of each alternative are suspended until later and will be reviewed in subsequent cognitive therapy steps.

Often clients will generate only variations of the same undesired outcome at first. Therapists ask clients to cover a full spectrum from best to worst, with many neutral, slightly positive, and slightly negative alternatives in between. Therapists often will write each alternative down on a marker board or a piece of paper to track them for clients. As clients describe their alternatives, therapists look for any aspect of the situation that remains unchanged in each alternative. Pointing the fixed detail out to the client and asking for alternatives that vary in that particular respect can be especially helpful. For example, a client might entertain possibilities of getting fired, promoted, or receiving an adequate job evaluation at work. The therapist might mention that all alternatives revolve around the client's current employer. The client could then be encouraged to generate alternatives in which he might decide not to work for his current employer. Outcomes such as quitting his job because he won the lottery or receiving a comparable job offer from another company suddenly become alternatives as well.

Other methods can help clients generate alternatives when they report feeling stuck or report they cannot think of any more. Group therapy settings are particularly useful for this purpose; group members offer a variety of possibilities while brainstorming alternatives to another client's specific anxious thought. In individual therapy settings, therapists might ask clients how an objective observer or an acquaintance might view the situation. As clients practice this step at home, they might ask significant others or friends for additional alternatives after generating as many as they can on their own. Craske and Barlow (2006a) instruct clients to list alternatives on a pie chart, with each alternative representing one possibility with an associated probability. However, this practice requires that clients first examine the relative likelihood of each alternative. Only those alternatives based on facts and evidence are included.

Traditionally, cognitive-behavioral therapists do subject automatic anxious thoughts to empirical examination before asking clients to generate alternatives. In our protocol, the generating alternatives technique is presented beforehand to promote cognitive flexibility from the outset. Generating alternatives in a brainstorming fashion without restrictions seems to enliven creative thinking processes. As clients see the array of possibilities in front of them, the uncertainty of their particular situation becomes apparent. Thus, clients are confronted with ambiguity early in the cognitive therapy process. This reversed sequence also reinforces the notion that a thought is only hypothetical. By generating alternatives freely from the beginning, clients experience first-hand that their thoughts are merely constructions of their minds. Indeed, many of our clients have described this effect. Generating alternatives immediately following identification of their anxious thoughts dramatically reduced associated emotional intensity. Distance between the thought and its emotional and behavioral impact was created from the start, enabling clients to approach the next step from a more objective stance than they otherwise would.

## Examining the Likelihood and Evidence

Most cognitive-behavioral therapists consider this technique the hallmark of cognitive therapy. Empirical examination of the original automatic anxious thought begins as therapists and clients explore its likelihood. Supporting as well as contrary evidence allows clients to compare objective probability to initial

subjective perceptions of probability. Likelihoods associated with alternative interpretations and predictions generated in the previous step are discussed as well. This
step directly corresponds to the first question of Beck and colleagues (1985),
"What's the evidence?" Evaluating the likelihood of a feared event is particularly
useful when clients are overestimating risks, a type of thinking Craske and Barlow
(2006b) termed "jumping to conclusions."

Therapists start by asking clients for a probability estimate of their automatic
anxious thought. If the thought represents a prediction about the future, what are
the chances the feared outcome will occur? If the thought represents an interpretation
of a past event, what is the likelihood the client's threatening interpretation is accurate? Clients estimate the probability with a percentage, where 0% reflects absolutely
no chance and 100% means absolute certainty. Therapists quickly point out that very
few life events come close to either extreme, again confronting clients with the uncertainty inherent in their situation. Typically clients report a probability that is less than
100 yet seems inflated to the therapist. In these cases, therapists remind clients that a
state of anxiety as well as a general tendency to feel anxious can make threatening
events seem more likely than they actually are. Indeed, Borkovec, Hazlett-Stevens,
and Diaz (1999) found that the feared outcomes reflected in college students' worry
happened only 32% of the time, suggesting an overestimation of probability in most
cases. In a smaller sample of clients diagnosed with GAD, these authors found that
only 15% of feared events actually turned out badly.

Therapists next question clients about the evidence upon which their likelihood
judgment was based. Questions such as "How do you know that [specific automatic
anxious thought] could happen" or "What leads you to think that [specific automatic anxious thought] is likely?" can be used. Often such questions will reveal a
circular type of reasoning in which the emotional intensity or severity of the anxiety
experienced has become the primary evidence of likelihood. Therapists remind clients that such emotional impact could be the result of the automatic thought and is
not factual evidence of its likelihood. The inflated subjective probability of an anxious thought often stems from the logical error of misconstruing feelings as evidence, a cognitive style known as "emotional reasoning."

Therapists continue to probe for any facts, actual events, or other concrete pieces
of information that may shed light on the feared situation's likelihood. Often a past
history or record of similar events can be examined. Questions such as "What has
happened before in similar situations?" or "Has [specific automatic anxious
thought] ever happened before?" might be helpful. Therapists then inquire about
any similarities or differences between previous events and the current situation. In
an example of a client worried about getting fired, the therapist would ask about
past job evaluations and any specific comments others have made about the client's
work performance. Importantly, therapists specifically should ask about any evidence to the contrary. Evidence in support of threat interpretations or feared outcomes is much more accessible than evidence that contradicts or otherwise does not
support the anxious thought. Therapists might bring this bias to clients' attention,
showing how clients often favor or "filter" evidence for their original anxious conclusion while "filtering out" or overlooking evidence against it. Other common

client biases include "overgeneralization" in which clients draw broad conclusions from isolated events and "mind reading" in which clients assume how other people are thinking or feeling. When therapists suspect clients are placing too much weight on a single piece of evidence, they can share their observations with clients and query for additional evidence. When clients rely on assumptions about the internal experiences (e.g., thoughts, feelings, motivations) of other people, therapists can identify these assumptions as such and ask about any factual evidence.

During this process therapists pose Socratic questions to clients as much as possible, resisting any urges to answer these questions for clients. Therapists also might feel tempted to state the logical conclusion at the end of a series of pointed questions for their clients. However, clients benefit most when they generate such conclusions themselves. Thus, therapists guide clients through a new process of empirical evaluation rather than attempt to argue clients away from their anxious thoughts. Clients come up with their own conclusions based on new information they had not considered previously. With enough examples of therapist-guided Socratic questioning in session, clients learn to ask the same types of questions themselves during assigned worry periods.

After examining surrounding factual evidence, therapists revisit initial probability estimates and invite clients to adjust their estimate based on any new considerations. Therapists also acknowledge that neither the client nor the therapist can determine an exact probability. Clients are only searching for their best estimate based on facts they have. By emphasizing that likelihood judgments are only estimates, therapists again bring the inherent uncertainty of the situation to clients' attention. Even the probability itself of an event is at least somewhat ambiguous. In our laboratory, chronic worriers chose gamble tasks with a known probability of winning more often than nonanxious participants did (Ritter & Hazlett-Stevens in preparation). Despite a greater *potential* for winning, high worriers often chose gambling scenarios in which the chances of winning were known instead of variable. Therapists should discuss any associated discomfort as clients discover the multitude of unknown factors that could impact their situation in unpredictable ways.

Therapists next guide clients through the alternatives generated in the previous step, estimating the likelihood and examining the evidence for each. Alternative interpretations or predictions can be evaluated in the same way the specific anxious thought was. Ideally the list of alternatives will encompass the gamut of probabilities, with most alternatives falling in the moderate likelihood range. Therapists point out how only a few alternatives are found on either extreme, none of which are completely zero or 100% likely. This practice further reinforces the uncertainty inherent in daily life. As clients see the range of probabilities, they are able to appreciate the complexity of the situation further.

After therapists and clients have examined as much available evidence as possible in session, they design an empirical test of the specific anxious thought. During the previous discussion, therapists are on the lookout for any unknown pieces of information clients could ascertain between sessions. Such "behavioral experiments" are conducted in much the same fashion as experimental research: (1) the original hypothesis reflected in the anxious thought is explicated, (2) clients execute an exact behavior to collect necessary information, and (3) possible conclusions are reviewed based on the outcome of the experiment. Therapists and clients collaborate on a specific task clients can perform between sessions that would reveal important information about the situation. For example, the client predicting to be fired at her next work evaluation might decide to approach her boss for feedback. A specific plan of action is crucial to the design of behavioral experiments. Clients should state exactly what they intend to do and what they will say to the other person beforehand. Therapists work with clients to clarify intended behaviors and guide clients toward options expected to elicit useful information without causing unintended negative impacts. If the behavioral experiment involves an interpersonal interaction, therapists and clients can role play likely conversations beforehand in session.

One final way clients can gather objective evidence is to track the actual outcomes reflected in automatic anxious thoughts. Worries representing future predictions are evaluated objectively once the feared events have occurred. Rather than discounting less threatening outcomes as they occur, clients are encouraged to track each eventual outcome systematically. During each worry period, clients review each specific anxious thought recorded previously. For each future prediction, has an actual outcome taken place yet? If so, clients compare what actually happened to the feared outcome predicted. Factual details involving the environment as well as client coping behavior should be considered. Similar to the experiment described by Borkovec et al. (1999), clients judge whether the actual outcome was better than, worse than, or comparable to their prediction. If the predicted event indeed happened, clients determine whether they coped better or worse than expected or as they expected. This assignment treats worrisome thoughts themselves as empirical investigations. Predicted outcomes are monitored systematically so that objective evidence of typical worries can be collected over time. As clients track worry outcomes, they accumulate an accurate body of evidence for use with later anxious thoughts.

Each day during the worry period, clients practice examining the likelihood and evidence as they reach the third column on the Thought Tracking Form. As modeled in session, clients estimate the likelihood of their automatic anxious thought and list all factual evidence both for and against it, including results from any behavioral experiments. Clients examine all evidence carefully, adjusting their initial likelihood estimate as needed. Clients then go back and estimate the likelihood of each alternative listed in the previous column. Before ending each worry period, clients review previous automatic anxious thoughts for worry outcome monitoring.

## Decatastrophizing

Although clients often overestimate the probability of feared events, some degree of possibility that the feared event could occur does exist. Clients also tend to overestimate the impact and severity of feared events should they occur, a type of anxious thinking Craske and Barlow (2006b) labeled "blowing things out of proportion." Decatastrophizing helps clients view unwanted events as manageable and questions views that they would be unable to cope with adversity. The previous step, examining the likelihood and evidence, challenges the first half of the standard anxious thought of Beck et al. (1985): "Something bad is going to happen." Decatastrophizing addresses the second half, "that I won't be able to handle." This technique corresponds to the third cognitive therapy question (Beck et al. 1985), "So what if it happens?" Clients discover that even if a particular feared event was certain to occur, its impact and any resulting events still remain uncertain. Clients struggling with GAD tend to report poor confidence in their problem-solving abilities (Ladouceur et al. 1998) as well as fears of incompetence and failure (Hazlett-Stevens & Craske, 2003b). The decatastrophizing technique encourages clients to follow their worries through to conclusion, considering the actual impact of undesired outcomes as well as how they would cope.

The term "decatastrophizing" is based on the observation that anxious clients often "catastrophize" the meaning of unwanted events. This tendency is reflected in statements such as "If [automatic anxious thought] happened, that would be terrible." Similar words suggesting a catastrophe such as "awful," "insufferable," "dreadful" and "disastrous" are common. To "de"-catastrophize, clients suppose the unwanted event in fact occurred. The first purpose of this practice is for clients to examine possible consequences other than the cascade of negative events assumed to follow. Second, clients examine how they would respond to the feared situation, realizing that they could cope with difficult situations and any associated emotion. Unlike usual worry, clients face their feared outcome and accept the worst case scenario as a possibility.

Therapists introduce this technique asking clients to suppose the anxious thought actually happened. What exactly would happen next? Therapists probe for any environmental and intrapersonal consequences clients envision as a result the feared event. Environmental consequences could include negative judgments of other people, loss of work, or financial ruin. Intrapersonal consequences might involve feeling like a failure, embarrassment, or suffering a painful loss. Catastrophic worry often involves a series of specific events in which each one is a condition of the other. Clients are rarely aware of the complex chain of negative events they assume would occur after the feared event. Therapists can help clients make such worry chains explicit with the downward arrow technique. The client's response to the initial question, "What if [anxious thought] actually happened?" is immediately followed by a similar question such as "What would happen then?" The therapist writes each subsequent response underneath an arrow pointing downward until the client cannot think of any more consequences. Consider the following hypothetical example of a client worried about losing her job.

Therapist:   Let's look at your automatic anxious thought "I will lose my job" a bit further. Now that we've examined the evidence and considered the likelihood, let's pretend for a moment this actually happened. What if you did lose your job…what exactly would happen next?

Client:        Well, I wouldn't be able to pay my bills that month.
Therapist:     And what would that lead to?
Client:        I'd get evicted from my apartment.
Therapist:     What would happen next?
Client:        I would have to live on the street.
Therapist:     And then what?
Client:        I don't know…I'd be lonely, scared, and miserable.

As the client answered each therapist question during this downward arrow technique, the therapist recorded each response. This resulted in the following diagram:

I will lose my job
↓
Wouldn't pay bills
↓
Evicted from apartment
↓
Live on the street
↓
Lonely, scared, miserable

Therapist:     Okay [showing client written responses]…here's what you're assuming would happen if you lost your job. Each time you think of losing your job, you seem to envision yourself homeless and destitute, living alone out on the street. It's as if you equate losing your current job with living homeless the rest of your life. How does this fit with your experience?
Client:        Yeah, I guess I am thinking that way…I never looked at it like this before.
Therapist:     Often this kind of catastrophic thinking is completely out of our awareness. That's why it can be useful to write each step down to examine objectively. Notice how each step in your worry chain is contingent upon the previous event. Every single step would have to happen before you become homeless, alone, and miserable.

At our University of Nevada, Reno program, we developed an expanded version of the standard downward arrow procedure that integrates decatastrophizing with the previous two cognitive therapy techniques. Once the client's worry chain is depicted with the original downward arrow technique, the therapist asks the client to generate at least two alternatives for each line. Clients estimate the probability of each worry chain line and are encouraged to select alternatives they believe are most likely to occur. These alternatives are written next to the original response generated during the first downward arrow exercise. Sometimes the therapist will repeat the downward arrow technique using new alternatives, allowing clients to see where else their feared event might lead. Eventually clients have a visual aid showing the complexity of possible events. This practice further reveals the uncertainty inherent in the situation even if the original feared event were certain to occur. In the above example, the client generated two alternatives to the second line, "wouldn't pay bills." The first, "would borrow money from parents to pay bills until I get a new job" and the second alternative,

"I would go back to school and apply for financial aid" both represented outcomes to losing her job other than not paying her bills. Neither alternative led to the subsequent consequences of eviction and homelessness.

Therapists also raise the possibility that the undesired event could lead to an unanticipated "fortunate" event. In our University of Nevada treatment program, we illustrate this point with a well-known Chinese folktale first incorporated into GAD treatment by Thomas Borkovec. This story of a farmer whose horse ran away appears in Watts (1975):

> That evening the neighbors gathered to commiserate with him since this was such bad luck. He said, "May be." The next day the horse returned, but brought with it six wild horses, and the neighbors came exclaiming at his good fortune. He said, "May be." And then, the following day, his son tried to saddle and ride one of the wild horses, was thrown, and broke his leg. Again the neighbors came to offer their sympathy for the misfortune. He said, "May be." The day after that, conscription officers came to the village to seize young men for the army, but because of the broken leg the farmer's son was rejected. When the neighbors came in to say how fortunately everything had turned out, he said, "May be." (Watts 1975, p. 31)

Hearing this story often helps clients see that a "bad" outcome sometimes leads to desirable opportunities they never considered. Therapists ask clients what this tale might mean for them, reinforcing the notion that no single event or outcome can truly be judged. Life's events unfold upon each other in unpredictable ways. Clients are encouraged to share their own "May be" story, in which an event considered unfortunate at the time actually led to something for which they are now quite grateful.

The second purpose of decatastrophizing is for clients to recognize their own coping resources. As seen in the above example, generating alternatives to worry chain consequences often prompts clients to consider what they might do. Clients begin to see they would have an array of behavioral responses if their feared event occurred. Feelings of helplessness tend to dissipate as clients articulate specific actions they would take to cope with the feared event. Therapists ask simple questions such as "What exactly would you do?" or "How would you cope with that situation?" to direct clients' attention toward adaptive coping behavior. Clients expressing difficulty are asked how they have coped with similar situations in the past. Eventually clients view themselves as capable of responding to difficult situations rather than victims of consequence.

Decatastrophizing requires clients to discuss the potential catastrophes associated with their feared outcomes. For this reason, this cognitive therapy technique resembles imaginal exposure therapies, although clients are facing only hypothetical events rather than actual past events. Nevertheless, clients may report extreme distress during these discussions, much as clients experience distress confronting phobic stimuli during exposure therapy. Therapists must be careful not to minimize the impact of tragic events. Therapists also should avoid invalidating any feelings of grief or despair that naturally would follow such tragic events. On the other hand, therapists can help clients appreciate that such events have not actually occurred. Clients cannot fully experience and process painful primary emotion when the event in question is merely hypothetical. Therapists therefore agree that truly tragic events such as losing a loved one would lead to significant emotional pain and suffering if such an event occurred. However, assertions that clients would never recover or would be unable to cope with such adversity can be examined. In addition, therapists can guide clients through a cost-benefit analysis of worrying about remote potential catastrophes simply because such events are possible. Disadvantages such as chronic tension are weighed against any perceived advantages. Clients convinced that worry about unlikely tragic events serves an adaptive function might benefit from further examination of their worry beliefs. Such beliefs about the need to worry as well as other fundamental assumptions and core beliefs are described next.

## Core Beliefs About the Self, the World, and the Future

The techniques described above teach new responses to the cognitive component of anxiety spirals. As clients practice identifying and challenging their automatic anxious thoughts, they develop yet another coping skill to replace habitual anxious responding. However, automatic anxious thoughts theoretically stem from fundamental views that have developed over the course of the individual's experiential history. Unless these core beliefs are also addressed, automatic anxious thoughts and threat interpretation biases will continue to appear. Thus, cognitive therapy also involves identification and restructuring of underlying beliefs about the self, the world (including other people), and the future (Beck et al. 1979). Individuals experiencing chronic worry and GAD tend to view themselves as incompetent, prone to failure, and unable to cope with adversity. Fundamental beliefs that the world is an unsafe and dangerous place lead to frequent states of hypervigilance. Not surprisingly, the uncertainty of the future is also perceived as threatening. As therapists and clients work together challenging automatic anxious thoughts, they begin to recognize any recurrent worry themes. Therapists soon discover the hidden meaning of feared events and associated underlying core beliefs. Decatastrophizing specific anxious thoughts can reveal deep fears of failure, avoidance of painful emotion, or core beliefs of the self as "not good enough" or unlovable. Many core beliefs are inherently interpersonal in nature, reflecting fears of rejection, disapproval, loneliness, or isolation. Once identified, these underlying beliefs can be examined with the cognitive therapy techniques described in the previous section. In addition, role play and other experiential therapy techniques help restructure self-defeating core beliefs.

### *Common Core Beliefs*

Many maladaptive expectations, assumptions, and rules associated with GAD stem from a fundamental negative view of the self. In particular, Beck et al. (1985) proposed that most daily life situations are perceived as threatening by individuals with

GAD "because 'inadequate' performance makes him feel constantly vulnerable to negative evaluation and rejection" (p. 101). These authors described the self-concept in GAD as ineffectual and therefore unable to cope with the demands of ordinary life. Subsequent research indeed found that views of the self as incompetent, inadequate, and vulnerable to failure were linked to excessive worry and GAD. Vasey and Borkovec (1992) studied the nature and content of worry chains with a systematic interview procedure based on the decatastrophizing cognitive therapy technique. Compared to a nonanxious comparison group, college students endorsing chronic worry generated more catastrophizing steps in their worry chains and reported increased distress over the course of the interview. In the subsequent content analysis, a greater proportion of chronic worriers' worry chain responses were categorized as representing "failure or ineffectiveness" when compared to nonanxions participant responses. In a similar investigation (Davey & Levy 1998), independent raters coded worry chain responses for "feelings of personal inadequacy." Trait worry, as measured by the Penn State Worry Questionnaire (PSWQ; Meyer, Miller, Metzger, & Borkovec 1990), was positively correlated with the number of steps generated as well as with personal inadequacy ratings. Hazlett-Stevens and Craske (2003b) conducted similar interviews with college students endorsing full GAD diagnostic criteria and a nonanxious comparison group. Based on the notion that the final interview step most likely reflected core underlying fears, only the endpoints of participant worry chains were coded for content. Among the participants with GAD, fears of negative emotion and fears of failure or ineffectiveness were coded most frequently. No group differences were found for fears of negative emotion. However, participants with GAD generated a greater proportion of failure or ineffectiveness responses than nonanxious participants did. Thus, clients suffering from GAD may hold deep-seated beliefs that they are fundamentally incompetent. Variants include believing the self to be inferior, "not good enough," inept, or unworthy of success.

Such entrenched views can originate from a variety of developmental circumstances, including cold or overly critical parents, overprotective parenting, or insecure parent-child attachment. One particular type of caregiver relationship was reported frequently by individuals with GAD: a "role-reversed/enmeshed" relationship (Cassidy 1995; Schut, Pincus, Castonguay, Bedics, et al. 1997). That is, as children, individuals with GAD perceived themselves as responsible for taking care of their primary caregiver. Thus, some clients indeed may have experienced actual circumstances in which they were not well-equipped to handle daily life situations. Negative views of the self might develop from a variety of childhood experiences in which an individual experienced him or herself as inadequate or incapable of coping with life situations.

Core beliefs about the self have crucial interpersonal implications. If the self is inadequate, inept, incompetent, or otherwise flawed, then other people ultimately will reject and disapprove. Individuals therefore might expect that others eventually will find oneself unworthy of love or acceptance. Fears of disapproval are often traced back to childhood relationships with caregivers or other important people in which love, approval, and acceptance felt contingent upon successful performance rather than given freely and unconditionally. In adulthood, such core beliefs about others make trust and intimacy difficult to attain, even in significant interpersonal relationships. When clients act upon maladaptive expectations of others, they create self-fulfilling prophecies. The other person is bound to disappoint as rigid relationship rules are violated. In addition, clients' own interpersonal behavior aimed at warding off disapproval and rejection often results in the exact opposite effect. As clients behave in ways expected to gain others' approval, they avoid truly intimate behaviors such as self-disclosure and authentic emotional expression. The resulting interpersonal disconnect only strengthens original fears of rejection and core beliefs that the self is not worthy of acceptance "as is." Genuine feelings of loneliness and unhappiness naturally follow. For this reason, Michelle Newman, Louis Castonguay, and Thomas Borkovec target maladaptive interpersonal behavior patterns directly in their newly developed "interpersonal/emotional processing" (I/EP) treatment for GAD (Newman, Castonguay, Borkovec, & Molnar 2004).

Other aspects of the external world are often viewed as threatening. Exaggerated beliefs that the world is dangerous and unpredictable may have developed from early circumstances that were indeed quite threatening. Not surprisingly, individuals with GAD reported significantly more past traumatic events than nonanxious comparison groups (Roemer, Molina, Litz, & Borkovec 1997). More subtle life experiences might play a role as well. For example, inconsistent caregiver behavior can leave children feeling unsafe and unprotected. External events therefore are experienced as unpredictable and uncontrollable, leading to views of the world as inherently unsafe in the absence of any life-threatening event. Role-reversed relationships in which children are charged with caring for an ill or depressed adult might be experienced as threatening if the adult does not reliably attend to the child's basic needs. Many similar life circumstances in which the outside world was experienced as unsafe could contribute to core beliefs that the world contains too many unanticipated dangers.

A view of the self as incapable of coping with adversity coupled with a view of the world as inherently dangerous result in negative views of the future. The uncertainty of the future seems overwhelming because upcoming threats cannot always be predicted and prevented. Negative beliefs about uncertainty itself also develop. Such "intolerance of uncertainty" appears unique to excessive worry; the relationship between intolerance of uncertainty and worry was not explained by links between worry and symptoms of anxiety or depression (see Dugas & Robichaud 2007 for a review). For this reason, the GAD treatment developed by Dugas and colleagues directly targets beliefs that uncertainty is harmful and helps clients become more tolerant of the future's uncertainties. Core beliefs that the uncertainty of the future cannot be tolerated reflect unrealistic demands that life should be completely predictable.

## Identifying and Examining Core Beliefs

Clients are rarely aware of the core beliefs driving their worry and anxiety. Given the emotional nature of these beliefs, many clients actively avoid examining them and associated past experiences. Therapists begin to identify clients' particular core beliefs as they challenge automatic anxious thoughts. Worry themes often emerge from the content of automatic thoughts as well as client responses to Socratic questions. The downward arrow exercise used for decatastrophizing often reveals core belief material near the bottom of the worry chain. Feared internal consequences, such as feeling difficult emotion or negative self-evaluation, can alert therapists to negative beliefs about the self or others. Therapists also can ask clients about core beliefs directly. Clients review Thought Tracking Form entries looking for any recurrent themes that may reflect underlying negative beliefs about themselves, the world, and the future. Therapist questions such as "What would it mean to you if [automatic anxious thought] occurred?" can lead to a fruitful discussion of core beliefs as well.

Once identified, core beliefs can be challenged with the same logical analysis method used to examine the evidence of automatic anxious thoughts. Core beliefs about the self can be examined by asking clients to define terms such as "failure," "success," or "loser." Such global labels often reflect specific characteristics or skills. Nevertheless, clients perceive such isolated instances as evidence of a larger negative view of themselves. Negative core beliefs about the self often appear as faulty causal attributions. That is, clients assume their incompetence caused certain unwanted events, thereby providing further "evidence" of their inadequacy. Similar to the cognitive style associated with depression (Abramson, Seligman, & Teasdale 1978), clients often make internal, stable, and global attributions about negative events. When an undesirable event does occur, clients may attribute its cause to some *internal* factor within themselves rather than external forces beyond their control. This internal factor is believed to be permanent and unchangeable, or *stable*. Lastly, clients consider these internal factors broad or *global*, expected to apply across many situations and life domains. When clients explain disappointing events to themselves as resulting from internal, stable, and global factors, the subsequent risk for depression, helplessness, and hopelessness are high. Furthermore, maladaptive behavior such as withdrawal and avoidance typically result. Therapists therefore encourage clients to generate external, temporary, specific causal explanations for failures as well as internal causal attributions for successes. In addition, clients are reminded that events are rarely caused by only one single internal or external factor, revealing the complexity of many life situations.

Unreasonable expectations for perfection often emerge as clients share their rigid personal rules with therapists. Karen Horney (1950) referred to these rules as the "tyranny of shoulds." Common examples include "I should never make mistakes," "I should never need help from other people," and "I should always work at optimal levels of productivity." As clients evaluate their self-imposed standards of perfection, therapists help them adjust rigid rules into more flexible expectations of themselves. Unrealistic views of control over the external world are also common. Clients suffering from GAD often endorse beliefs that they are responsible for everything that happens to themselves and to others. Such clients believe they should be able to exercise complete control over their environment, and then inevitably feel guilty or incompetent when they cannot. Clients also may entertain self-defeating views at the opposite extreme, feeling helpless and entirely out of control.

Balanced perspectives involve accepting that many external factors cannot be controlled and that each individual is responsible for himself or herself. Clients are therefore accountable for taking care of themselves and for choosing how they behave, but they are not responsible for the problems and challenges other people face. Clients learn to accept circumstances and possibilities beyond their control while taking charge over their own behavior in deliberate and adaptive ways.

Core beliefs about the self sometimes involve negative beliefs about internal emotional experience. Many clients believe they should not or could not bear uncomfortable or painful emotions. In the experiment described above (Hazlett-Stevens & Craske 2003b), we found that both GAD and nonanxious comparison groups frequently reported some type of negative emotional experience in the final step of their worry chains. However, fear and avoidance of painful emotion may be pronounced in GAD. Borkovec and Roemer (1995) conducted a survey investigation of the perceived functions of worry with individuals diagnosed with GAD, anxious individuals endorsing only somatic symptom GAD diagnostic criteria, and a nonanxious comparison group. Participants with full GAD rated the belief that worry serves as a distraction from even more emotional topics more highly than participants in both comparison groups. Perhaps some individuals with GAD have indeed suffered more emotional pain from past experiences than less worried people have. Regardless of past circumstances, primary emotional experience can be tolerated and processed. Therapists might educate clients about the adaptive function of emotions, in which basic emotional reactions provide useful feedback about our environment. Although basic emotions such as hurt and sadness are uncomfortable and even painful, they do not destroy people. Other emotions such as embarrassment also can be tolerated. Emotions fluctuate over time and are not static. Intense feelings experienced at one point in time do not simply remain at high levels indefinitely. Clients are encouraged to experiment with allowing uncomfortable emotions to test core beliefs that intense emotions are unbearable.

Unrealistic expectations of others also result from core beliefs. When rigid rules and perfectionist standards are applied to other people, disappointment eventually follows. Assumptions about the motives of significant others can be challenged when their behavior was perceived as unfair. Some clients hold hidden expectations that if they sacrifice their own needs to care for others, they will ultimately receive appreciation, affection, and love in return. Maladaptive interpersonal behaviors include trying to change other people and intrusive care-taking. In addition, clients may avoid asserting themselves clearly and directly yet become resentful when others do not anticipate their needs. Self-disclosure of innermost thoughts, feelings, and hopes are also avoided due to core beliefs that significant others may disapprove. As maladaptive expectations and behaviors are examined, clients learn to accept imperfection in others and assume responsibility for asserting their own preferences, desires, and needs.

Finally, core beliefs about the future and fears of uncertainty are restructured. Beliefs that life should not involve risk or that risks should always be known are examined. Therapists challenge an exaggerated need for certainty by encouraging clients to evaluate their own behavior when demanding complete certainty. Most clients will recognize that they fail to act while trying to achieve greater certainty. Dugas and Robichaud (2007) recommended that therapists discuss the role of intolerance of uncertainty in excessive worry, identify how clients try to eliminate uncertainty in their daily lives, and assign "tolerating uncertainty experiments" related to clients' worry themes.

Clients continue to examine core beliefs during between-session worry periods. Once these beliefs have been identified and examined in therapy sessions, clients identify which core belief(s) may underlie each automatic anxious thought recorded on the Thought Tracking Form. After working an automatic anxious thought through the first four steps, clients reflect upon any fundamental views of themselves, the world, and the future that might be responsible for the thought. Clients then walk the core belief through the previous cognitive therapy steps, drawing from previous therapy discussions.

## Additional Strategies for Restructuring Core Beliefs

Examining core beliefs with traditional cognitive therapy techniques can yield significant therapeutic gains. When core beliefs become less and less believable to clients, their impact is greatly reduced. For some clients, however, logical analysis of the evidence is only a starting point. In addition to Socratic questioning, therapists can ask clients to role play responses to another person's negative core beliefs. Clients pretend that a friend has just disclosed having the same core belief the client identified in session. As the therapist plays the role of the troubled friend, the client challenges the core belief from a compassionate stance.

Some cognitive-behavioral therapists have begun to integrate experiential therapy techniques into their practice. Goldfried (1996) demonstrated the "two-chair technique" to address a client's core belief that her significant other would reject her if she revealed her true thoughts and feelings to him. Two chairs were positioned facing each other in the therapy session. Each side of this issue was represented by a different chair, and the client argued each opposing side from each respective chair. The client first spoke as her true self, expressing genuine feelings about her significant other and explaining why she would like to open up to him. She then switched chairs and responded as the part of herself afraid her significant other would not accept her true self and would eventually leave her. This dialogue continued as the client argued each side from each chair with the therapist prompting her throughout. As this process continued, the client appeared to experience associated emotions more intensely. Eventually the client was able to express her authentic desires for the relationship. During her subsequent discussion with the therapist, she decided that she would disclose this fear to her significant other and tell him how much she cares for him. Goldfried adapted this experiential technique so that the emotional meanings underlying cognitive material could be accessed and processed in treatment. From this perspective, CBT might be enhanced by clinical attention to these emotional meanings rather than an exclusive focus on the intellectual meaning of cognition (Samilov & Goldfried 2000). Furthermore, effective cognitive restructuring is considered most likely when the cognition is "hot," having just occurred naturally with its associated emotional salience. Indeed, Newman and colleagues (2004) integrated experiential techniques into their I/EP treatment for GAD. Problematic relationship patterns are addressed by exploring past and current relationships as well as interactions between the therapist and client. Clients practice new interpersonal behaviors between therapy sessions. In addition, associated emotional experience is encouraged during therapy sessions with various emotional deepening techniques, including the two-chair technique described above. As discussed in Chap. 2, preliminary research suggested that I/EP may improve the efficacy of traditional CBT for individuals diagnosed with GAD (Newman et al.).

Finally, therapists and clients explore the origins of the core belief. Therapists ask clients to reflect upon what developmental experiences may have led to the belief. Many circumstances described above, such as overly critical or overprotective parents, might be identified. Other common examples include a parent who failed to protect the child from actual danger or a parent who relied on the child to care for them, thereby creating a role-reversed relationship. Core beliefs often weaken as clients understand how their experience has taught them to view themselves as incompetent and the world and future as threatening. These discussions about the original source of the belief also can lead to "empty chair" experiential exercises (Greenberg, Rice, & Elliott 1996). In their I/EP treatment for GAD, Newman et al. (2004) apply this particular exercise when clients have unresolved feelings toward another person. Clients imagine the parent or other significant person sitting across from them in an empty chair. Clients express their true feelings about the situation and the other person while speaking in the present tense with first-person language (e.g., "I feel …"). As clients address the parent or other influential person, they learn to tolerate and to process their unresolved primary emotions. Such emotional processing tends to loosen previously learned core beliefs. A variation of this technique involves asking the client to write a letter to the other person, expressing associated feelings and detailing the impact the other person's actions had on the client. The client writes the letter between sessions and then shares the letter with the therapist in the subsequent therapy session. These letters are intended for therapeutic purposes and therefore are rarely sent or otherwise shared with the other person.

## Meta-Cognitive Worry Beliefs

Among individuals with GAD, core beliefs reflecting Beck's "cognitive triad" can lead to specific beliefs about the nature and function of worry known as meta-cognitive worry beliefs. Clients often believe that frequent or constant worry is necessary to cope with impending threat. If left unaddressed, such "positive" worry beliefs could undermine all other therapy techniques. Clients are unwilling to implement worry reduction procedures faithfully when they are also motivated to worry for perceived benefit. On the other hand, worry about worry itself, or meta-worry, stems from "negative" worry beliefs, or fears of the perceived deleterious consequences of chronic worry. Negative worry beliefs might prevent clients from engaging in self-monitoring and cognitive therapy assignments due to fears of increased worry and anxiety. Both types of meta-cognitive worry beliefs can be examined using the cognitive therapy techniques described above. Clients practice identifying and examining these worry beliefs when they reach the fifth Thought Tracking Form column during each subsequent worry period.

## Positive Worry Beliefs

When clients view themselves as incompetent and view the future as threatening, they often consider worry a needed means for coping with future threats. Based on this clinical observation, Borkovec and Roemer (1995) asked clients participating in a GAD psychotherapy outcome investigation if they perceived any benefits or advantages to worry despite its associated distress. Borkovec and Roemer then developed a brief questionnaire reflecting the six major themes that emerged from client responses: (1) Worry helps motivate me to get things done that I need to get done, (2) Worrying is an effective way to problem-solve, (3) If I worry about something, when something bad does happen, I'll be better prepared for it, (4) If I worry about something, I am more likely to actually figure out how to avoid or prevent something bad from happening, (5) Worrying about most of the things that I worry about is a way to distract myself from even more emotional things, things that I don't want to think about, (6) Although it may not actually be true, it feels like if I worry about something, the worrying makes it less likely that something bad will happen. In the research investigation that followed, participants diagnosed with GAD as well as anxious and nonanxious comparison groups without GAD all endorsed the same three beliefs most: worry helps avoid or prevent bad outcomes, worry helps prepare for something bad when it does happen, and worry is an effective way to solve problems. As described above, another worry belief was endorsed more by clients with GAD than both comparison groups: worry distracts from more emotional topics. Thus, while worry indeed may function to avoid feared emotional experience among clients with GAD, other beliefs about its utility to cope with external situations are quite common.

Beliefs about the adaptive functions of worry could originate from an accumulation of past experiences in which feared events did not occur. Through the process of negative reinforcement, worry becomes more likely each time the absence of an unwanted outcome happens to follow. Faulty causal attributions about worry (i.e., "The bad thing didn't happen *because* I worried about it") eventually develop. Worry soon becomes a superstitious covert behavior clients are afraid to abandon. Indeed, Hazlett-Stevens, Zucker, and Craske (2002) found that college students endorsing full GAD diagnostic criteria believed that thoughts directly impact the likelihood of unwanted external events more than a nonanxious comparison group did. Furthermore, in instances where worry is followed by the unwanted event, faulty causal attributions still could be made about the resulting impact (i.e., "I coped with the bad thing well *because* I was prepared by my worry" or "The bad thing wasn't as bad as it would have been had I not worried about it to prepare"). As therapists and clients discuss underlying positive worry beliefs, therapists can explain the concept of negative reinforcement and how it applies to worry. Clients learn why worry feels so necessary to them, why positive worry beliefs feel so true, and how strong superstitions about worry may have developed.

Therapists can help clients identify idiosyncratic positive worry beliefs simply by asking about them. Despite the unwanted anxiety and emotional distress, does the client also see any benefits to worrying? What advantages might clients see to worry even in light of its disadvantages? Another approach involves asking clients to imagine that worry was impossible. What if they couldn't worry? What would that be like? What might happen? Often clients will report a sudden spike in anxiety at the prospect of not being able to worry. Exploring why an automatic anxiety response just occurred can reveal any feared consequences associated with the absence of worry. In our protocol at the University of Nevada, we introduce the topic of positive worry beliefs with a written list of the six beliefs identified by Borkovec and Roemer (1995). Clients identify which worry beliefs fit best with their own experience. Therapists question whether any of the other worry beliefs also might apply. This method conveys that positive worry beliefs are common and can be understood even though these beliefs contradict clients' stated therapy goals. Clients therefore are less embarrassed to admit their positive worry beliefs and more willing to explore these beliefs in treatment.

As positive worry beliefs are identified, each can be examined for evidence using the same cognitive therapy techniques described above. If clients made causal attributions about their worry, therapists ask for alternative explanations. What reasons other than clients' worry could account for desirable outcomes? Perhaps the external feared event would not have occurred regardless of whether or not the client thought about it beforehand. Behavioral experiments also address perceived useful functions of worry. Clients can select a specific day or period of time when they worry as they typically would and then postpone their worry as often as possible on the following day. During each time period, clients carefully track the actual outcomes related to their worry topics. Clients and therapists then empirically examine whether fewer feared events occurred when clients worried and whether any events in question would have occurred anyway. Clients also are encouraged to reflect back on times in their lives when they worried less than they do now. Did threatening events happen more often? Sometimes clients recognize that they coped with daily life as well as or even better than they do now. If unwanted events did occur, would such events have happened anyway? Beliefs about the need to worry sometimes can be traced back to a major negative life event that coincidentally occurred when the client had not been worrying. In this case, beliefs that an absence of worry was responsible for the negative event can be challenged.

Clients also may believe they need to worry to manage their own behavior. Often clients describe that worry motivates them to accomplish important tasks. Worry has become a negative reinforcement strategy in which clients worry about accomplishing a task until its completion. Thus, temporary removal of an aversive worry state is the "reward" for the accomplishment. Therapists can redirect client efforts toward more adaptive behavioral management strategies. Clients can learn to motivate themselves with positive reinforcement contingencies in which clients reward themselves with something pleasant as they complete each work task. In addition to reducing associated emotional distress, positive reinforcement strategies reduce the likelihood of procrastination and therefore are ultimately more effective. Clients who believe worry enables them to solve problems can question exactly how their worry leads to adaptive behavior. Indeed, worry stems from the cognitive ability to anticipate future problems. However, such "worry" is constructive only when adaptive action follows. For this reason, clients identify concrete problems and take adaptive problem-solving action whenever possible during initial thought tracking. With practice, clients learn to discriminate between concrete problems with solutions under their control and vague concerns or unlikely events beyond their control.

Finally, all positive worry beliefs can be challenged with a cost-benefit analysis. Clients are asked to list all perceived advantages to worry as well as the perceived disadvantages. In addition to examining each perceived advantage as a hypothesis, therapists might probe for any unrecognized disadvantages. For example, the cumulative effects of chronic sleep disturbance and other GAD somatic symptoms might adversely affect clients' daily functioning. Worry consumes much attention and concentration, thereby distracting clients from important information available in the present moment. Clients might be able to identify an instance when they missed something important from the environment because they were preoccupied with worry. Furthermore, worry can carry interpersonal costs. Clients are often so invested in worrying to prevent threat that they underestimate any actual negative impact on others. Clients even may hold beliefs that worry enhances their relationships, believing that worry communicates love and caring to significant others. However, worry often prevents clients from perceiving others' needs accurately. Some clients discover that worry has become a means of getting attention from other people. Unless they express worry, other people will not take them seriously and recognize the issue as valid. Therapists help these clients search for more adaptive ways to express themselves and to communicate with others. Once all perceived advantages and disadvantages have been identified, clients might argue for and against worry using the same two-chair technique described for core beliefs.

## Negative Worry Beliefs

Clients often develop exaggerated beliefs about the harmful consequences of their worry. In his cognitive model of GAD, Wells (2004) proposed that meta-worry, or catastrophic worry about worry itself, stems from beliefs that worry is mentally, physically, or socially dangerous. Fears that worry could cause one to go crazy, lose touch with reality, or lose behavioral control are common. Related beliefs that worry is inherently uncontrollable also characterize GAD. According to this model, individuals worry about external events ("Type 1" worry) when they hold positive worry beliefs about its utility. If negative worry beliefs are also present, then "Type 2" worry, or worry about the Type 1 worry, will also result. Wells considers Type 2 worry (i.e., meta-worry) the more problematic worry because individuals respond with thought suppression and other thought control attempts. Such attempts increase associated emotional distress and paradoxically may increase intrusive thoughts and images. Indeed, two investigations examined the effects of worry immediately following exposure to a gruesome film (Butler, Wells, & Dewick 1995; Wells & Papageorgiou, 1995). In both studies, participants randomly assigned to worry demonstrated a greater frequency of distressing images over the subsequent three days compared to participants who engaged in imagery or other control tasks after viewing the film instead.

Wells (2004) therefore recommended that cognitive therapy primarily target negative worry beliefs. From this perspective, restructuring negative beliefs reduces not only meta-worry but also any counterproductive attempts to control worry. Emotional distress associated with Type 1 worry decreases as clients discover that such worry is not inherently harmful to them. Therapists empathize with the double-bind many individuals with GAD perceive. On the one hand, worry is viewed as necessary to prevent or to cope with impending threat. On the other hand, clients fear perceived consequences of worrying too much. Many of the genuine disadvantages of excessive worry described above can be reframed as a motivation to invest in therapy and to try new therapy behaviors. However, beliefs that worry will cause clients to lose control or go crazy, will make them seriously ill, or will result in rejection by others can be examined with the cognitive therapy techniques presented earlier in this chapter. Polarized views of worry as either "all bad" or "all good" can be broadened to a more flexible perspective. Are there instances in which worry might not be harmful or even may be productive? Worry stems from an adaptive ability to think ahead into the future. Sometimes thinking ahead can lead to effective problem solving, planning, and constructive behavior. Excessive and unproductive worry might contribute to somatic symptoms and emotional distress, but these effects are reversible with treatment do not cause permanent damage. Finally, beliefs that worry can never be controlled are restructured as clients practice postponing worry to a worry period.

## Establishing New Perspectives

Once clients have challenged automatic anxious thoughts and examined underlying beliefs, they can create new, more adaptive perspectives. The final column on the Thought Tracking Form prompts clients to revise their original anxious thought into a more balanced, flexible, and adaptive version. During later therapy sessions, therapists help clients adopt "preventive" beliefs that counter the core beliefs identified earlier. As clients practice this final step on the Thought Tracking Form during their scheduled worry periods, they develop their own coping self-statements. Clients eventually incorporate their cognitive therapy skills into daily life, applying new coping self-statements in response to anxiety spiral cues and stressful situations.

## Developing New Perspectives

In this final step, clients describe a new way of looking at the situation that is more balanced and flexible—yet less anxiety-provoking—than the original automatic anxious thought. Clients first review all new information generated during the previous cognitive therapy steps, and then summarize their main conclusions in one or two sentences. Clients incorporate any realizations made and objective evidence discovered that impacted them the most. Conclusions from cost-benefit analyses conducted for underlying core beliefs or worry beliefs are also included. New perspectives often take a larger context into account, reflecting the "bigger picture." These revised perspectives should be free of vague or abstract terms, assumptions, overgeneralizations, and rigid rules. Beck et al. (1985) recommended that clients convert major issues into minor concerns by expressing their desires as preferences instead of needs. These authors also directed clients toward perceptions of choice. That is, clients might continue to experience automatic thoughts but they can choose their responses to such thoughts and explore multiple perspectives. Although therapists provide guidance as clients generate new perspectives, clients must come up with their own perspectives which seem believable and make sense to them.

## Constructing Preventive Beliefs

In addition to creating new perspectives in response to automatic anxious thoughts, therapists and clients construct "preventive" beliefs. These beliefs counter previously identified core beliefs because they are flexible and appreciate complexity, unlike anxiety-provoking core beliefs. Preventive beliefs are intended to prevent subsequent overestimation of threat and underestimation of coping ability. Once clients and therapists develop a couple of preventive beliefs that address major concerns, clients are instructed to behave "as if" the preventive belief was valid and the previous core belief was not. For example, a client describing a core belief that he is inferior to other people might develop a preventive belief that overall comparisons between people realistically cannot be made. No valid unit of measurement exists to determine if one person is more worthy than another person. Each person has unique strengths and weakness; an individual's accomplishments simply reflect a series of choices and opportunities. If this client behaved according to the preventive belief instead of the core belief, he might pursue new employment opportunities, invite a woman out on a date, or ask his boss for a raise.

## *Application of Cognitive Strategies*

New perspectives and preventive beliefs are developed to promote adaptive behavior in general. Eventually clients also apply their new perspectives to specific anxiety cues as they occur in daily life. When clients detect an automatic anxious thought during regular self-monitoring, they respond with coping self-statements. That is, clients practice saying anxiety-reducing statements to themselves based on previous new perspectives and preventive beliefs. Clients tailor their coping self-statements to the particular situation at hand as a means of coping with the situation more effectively. Clients first practice their coping self-statements in session during the imaginal coping rehearsal procedure described in Chap. 7, self-control desensitization.

Clients sometimes are tempted to skip over previous steps and go directly to this final step, essentially bypassing the cognitive therapy process. Therapists should warn clients that such "short-cuts" to the final step are ineffective and even may backfire. Cognitive therapy is not simply replacing negative thoughts with positive thoughts. Meaningful therapeutic change results from effortful examination of the facts and generation of multiple perspectives. Unless clients earnestly do the work required in the previous steps, the new perspective will contain only general statements of reassurance without real value or meaning. Such empty platitudes (e.g., "Everything is going to be alright") lack many of the important characteristics described above. Therapists therefore caution clients against misuse of this final step as a self-reassurance strategy. Therapists explain how trying to reassure oneself can become a safety behavior that undermines treatment efforts, just as seeking reassurance from others can. Instead, clients must discover new perspectives for themselves and generate coping self-statements from within. New perspectives, preventive beliefs, as well as the specific coping self-statements generated from them, only have meaning after clients have worked through anxious thoughts and beliefs (see Client Handout 6.1).

## Chapter Summary

The cognitive therapy component described in this chapter was based largely on the work of Beck and colleagues (Beck et al. 1979, 1985). From this perspective, excessive anxiety results from maladaptive and inflexible threat interpretations. Clients often overestimate risks while underestimating their own ability to cope with life circumstances. Cognitive therapy techniques therefore teach clients to identify automatic anxious thoughts and to examine them objectively. Therapists pose Socratic questions to expose new information clients had not previously considered. Importantly, this Socratic questioning method guides clients toward discovery of their own new perspectives. In the case of GAD, cognitive therapy aims to expand client perspectives by revealing the complexity and ambiguity inherent in most life situations. As clients learn to appreciate complexity and to tolerate ambiguity, their cognitive flexibility also may increase. Eventually, clients apply new cognitive perspectives as another coping response to anxiety spiral cues.

Initial cognitive therapy procedures are introduced early in treatment. Therapists explain the rationale behind cognitive therapy and teach clients to identify automatic anxious thoughts. Clients then practice identifying automatic anxious thoughts as they naturally occur over the course of daily life. Each time worry is detected, clients record the specific anxious thought on a Thought Tracking Form. At that moment, clients remind themselves that their thought is only hypothetical and is not a fact. Clients then determine whether their anxious thought reflects a concrete problem for which they can take constructive action. If so, they shift their efforts to immediate action. If not, clients postpone the worry to a worry period and redirect their attention back to the present moment. Worry periods are scheduled times each day when clients review their worries and examine their anxious thoughts with cognitive therapy techniques.

Once clients have experienced some degree of mastery with these initial procedures, therapists teach clients to challenge their automatic anxious thoughts with three standard techniques. First, clients brainstorm for alternative interpretations or predictions. Clients generate as many different alternatives as they can, spanning a wide range of possibilities. Second, clients examine the likelihood of their automatic anxious thoughts and systematically examine the evidence both for and against them. Clients also compare evidence for their automatic anxious thoughts to evidence for any alternatives generated in the previous step. Third, clients decatastrophize automatic anxious thoughts by supposing feared events actually have occurred. Using an expanded version of the downward arrow technique, clients generate subsequent feared outcomes as well as alternative outcomes. Ways in which clients would cope with feared outcomes are explored as well. Each technique is represented by a column on the Thought Tracking Form, allowing clients to take each automatic anxious thought through this series of steps on their own during worry periods. Unlike other cognitive therapy protocols, we encourage clients to generate alternative interpretations or predictions up front before examining the likelihood and evidence of each. This sequence appears to facilitate creative and flexible thinking from the outset, and also seems to reinforce the concept that thoughts are only hypothetical.

Automatic anxious thoughts theoretically stem from underlying core beliefs about the self, other people, the external world, and the future. Meta-cognitive beliefs about worry itself also may fuel anxious cognition and behavior. As clients become adept identifying and challenging their specific automatic anxious thoughts, therapists next help them look for recurrent worry themes and underlying beliefs. Core beliefs include viewing the self as incompetent or otherwise flawed, viewing others as ultimately disapproving or rejecting, and viewing the external world and the future as threatening. Once identified, these core beliefs can be challenged with the same techniques described for automatic anxious thoughts. Additional experiential therapy techniques might provide a particularly effective way to loosen rigid, negative views of the self and of others. As clients become aware of the core beliefs underlying their automatic anxious thoughts, they record these beliefs on the Thought Tracking Form and examine them during subsequent worry periods between sessions.

Meta-cognitive beliefs about worry also should be identified and examined. In the case of positive worry beliefs, clients are convinced worry serves an adaptive function or otherwise provides some benefit. Negative worry beliefs are exaggerated fears about the harmful consequences of worry, such as worry causing one to "go crazy" or lose touch with reality. Both types of worry beliefs are common among individuals with GAD, leading to a perceived double-bind in which worry feels necessary yet ultimately could result in permanent damage. Both types of worry beliefs can undermine treatment efforts and should be challenged with the cognitive therapy techniques described above. For example, clients conduct behavioral experiments to test their theories about any perceived benefits of worry. Worry beliefs also can be subjected to cost-benefit analysis in which clients compare perceived advantages to any overlooked disadvantages.

Once automatic anxious thoughts and underlying beliefs have been restructured, clients create a new perspective that is more balanced and flexible than the original automatic anxious thought. New perspectives should seem believable and reasonable to clients yet incorporate the complexity and ambiguity inherent in the situation. Clients summarize their conclusions from the previous cognitive therapy steps and write a statement reflecting their new perspective in the final column of the Thought Tracking Form. Therapists and clients develop preventive beliefs that counter original core beliefs, and therapists encourage clients to act "as if" the preventive beliefs were more valid. Finally, clients generate brief coping self-statements to use as cognitive coping responses whenever automatic anxious thoughts are detected. Clients must work through cognitive restructuring steps before application of coping self-statements will be effective.

# Chapter 7
# Behavior Therapy and Exposure Strategies

The ultimate aim for most, if not all, psychotherapy is effective behavior change. Adaptive shifts in affect and cognition allow clients to try new behaviors. Clients soon become willing to approach previously avoided situations and to eliminate subtle safety behaviors associated with inflated perceptions of threat. Many clients naturally exhibit some adaptive behavior change as the interventions described in the previous chapters take effect. Nevertheless, therapists should systematically address any anxiety-promoting behavior, as even the most subtle forms of avoidance can maintain anxious disturbance.

Given the diffuse nature of the anxiety seen in GAD, clients may be completely unaware of their avoidance behavior. Unlike specific phobias with circumscribed feared stimuli, avoidance behavior associated with GAD can be difficult for clinicians to identify. Active avoidance—behavior executed to reduce anxiety—appears in the form of various subtle worry safety behaviors. Craske and colleagues examined worry monitoring records of nineteen clients diagnosed with GAD (Craske, Rapee, Jackel, & Barlow 1989). Over half (52.6%) of the worries recorded were associated with some sort of active avoidance behavior. Passive avoidance behavior—escape or withdrawal from feared situations or failure to approach them in the first place—also can present in subtle ways. Both forms of avoidance behavior can undermine treatment efforts by strengthening perceptions of threat. Clients attain immediate relief from avoidance behavior, but deprive themselves the opportunity to experience what would have happened and how they would have coped. Reductions in discomfort negatively reinforce the avoidance behavior, thereby increasing the likelihood of an avoidance response in future situations. For these reasons, therapists help clients identify and eliminate any anxiety-enhancing avoidance behavior.

The therapy techniques described in this chapter target the behavioral component of anxiety spirals directly. Clients learn to resist their habitual behavioral responses when they detect worry or other anxiety cues. Coping responses are deployed in place of safety behavior. Feared situations are identified so that clients can confront each between sessions. During therapy sessions, clients practice new responses with a coping imagery rehearsal procedure known as self-control desensitization. Finally, therapists encourage clients to engage in previously neglected activities which promote physical health and emotional well-being.

H. Hazlett-Stevens, *Psychological Approaches to Generalized Anxiety Disorder*,
doi: 10.1007/978-0-387-76870-0, © Springer Science + Business Media, LLC 2008

# Active Avoidance: Worry Safety Behavior

Many clients suffering from GAD have developed idiosyncratic worry-related behaviors as a means of coping with perceived threat. Any overt or covert action clients take to minimize the likelihood or impact of feared events can be considered active avoidance behavior. After therapists and clients identify specific worry safety behaviors, clients systematically resist urges to engage in each. If clients become overwhelmed, this response prevention intervention can be broken down into gradual steps. However, clients may not be willing to cease worry behavior unless they understand the underlying rationale. Therapists first ask clients how they believe worry safety behavior fuels their anxiety spirals. In the discussion that follows, therapists explain how this behavior increases perceptions of threat and prevents clients from learning first-hand what actually would have happened otherwise. Any client beliefs about the perceived protective function of their safety behavior should be addressed before home practice assignments are made. Until clients appreciate that worry-related behavior perpetuates anxious symptoms in the long term, they most likely will hesitate to follow therapists' response prevention instructions.

## *Identifying Worry Safety Behavior*

Clients already may have discovered specific worry safety behavior through the self-monitoring procedures described in Chap. 4. Therapists identify additional safety behavior by asking what clients do to feel safe when they are worried. Clients also might imagine a recent anxiety episode, describing each reaction as it occurred. This practice helps clients become aware of any behavioral habits they may have developed to reduce distress. If clients are unable to identify worry-related behavior in session, they carefully observe any mental or behavioral action taken in response to anxiety cues over the next week. In the following session, therapists ask about any specific behavior clients noticed as they detected worry. Therapists then review each prominent worry topic for any associated preventive action. Worry behaviors typically appear connected to the worry topic in a logical or predictable way. For example, clients worried about making mistakes will excessively check their work. Occasionally the worry behavior will seem random or superstitious, such as knocking on wood or counting.

Various kinds of checking behavior are common among individuals with GAD. Frequent repeated checking of documents or other written work may serve to catch any mistakes. Clients may repeatedly check scheduled appointment times to prevent missing meetings or other events. Sometimes worry-related checking behavior resembles that of individuals suffering from the doubting and checking type of OCD: clients who worry excessively about physical safety may repeatedly check that the door is locked or that the oven has been turned off. Clients worried about the safety of others may call loved ones frequently to check that they are safe. Many checking behaviors serve the purpose of providing clients with temporary reassurance that the feared event has been prevented or has not yet occurred. Other attempts to gain reassurance include asking trusted friends or family members for assurance that a feared event is unlikely or would be manageable. Clients also might seek reassurance or advice when making everyday decisions rather than trust their own judgments.

In addition to checking and reassurance-seeking, other worry safety behaviors attempt to prevent mistakes, failure, and the disapproval of others. Some clients may complete all work tasks themselves out of fear that delegating responsibilities to others will result in increased human error. Clients worried about work performance evaluations may work late or seek out a heavy workload. Similarly, others may over-prepare for work presentations or meetings to avoid the scrutiny of co-workers. Clients afraid of disappointing others might agree to extra work tasks or make commitments in their personal lives they otherwise would not. Some clients report mentally rehearsing a conversation ahead of time to prevent not knowing what to say and appearing foolish. One particular example reported by Brown, O'Leary, and Barlow (2001) involves frequent cleaning. Unlike clients who clean excessively due to contamination fears, some individuals with GAD keep certain home or office areas clean to prevent others from seeing messy or cluttered space. Clients afraid of being late often leave home much earlier than necessary for routine medical appointments. Worry behaviors intended to prevent physical harm include overprotective parenting practices to ensure the safety of children. Clients worried about their own safety may exhibit other forms of overly cautious behavior. As discussed in Chap. 6, even worry itself can be conceptualized as a covert safety behavior when clients hold positive worry beliefs about the need to worry.

## *Eliminating Worry Safety Behavior*

Once clients become aware of their own safety behavior, therapists encourage clients to refrain from the behavior each time they notice an urge. Clients instead practice an alternative coping response, such as a brief applied relaxation exercise. For clients with little worry safety behavior, these general response prevention instructions may suffice. Therapists follow up in subsequent sessions by asking about response prevention efforts and what actually happened when clients did not engage in worry safety behavior.

For many clients, however, a more systematic and gradual approach to response prevention is best. Therapists and clients identify specific instances and settings in which clients will attempt response prevention practice. After initial success, response prevention instructions are expanded to cover increasingly longer periods of time. In each therapy session, therapists review the previous home practice assignment. Clients describe their specific response prevention attempts and what happened regarding feared consequences. Therapists and clients then collaborate to decide upon the next home practice assignment for the following week. For example, a client who spends 2 hours each afternoon cleaning her living room and kitchen may select one particular day over the next week for response prevention practice. Instead of her regular cleaning that day, she could plan to go shopping during her usual cleaning time that afternoon and agree not to clean when she returns home until the following afternoon. After success with this initial assignment, response prevention on additional days could be assigned. Eventually, this client would limit her cleaning to a reasonable routine and resist acting upon the urge to clean when worried. In a second example, a client who calls her husband several times per day to check on his safety might refrain from calling in the morning and call only two or three prescheduled times each afternoon. She would instruct her husband not to answer any questions about his safety or otherwise provide reassurance during these calls. In the subsequent week, she would reduce these phone calls further to one per day. Eventually the client could try an entire week without calling at all. Finally, this client would plan only to call her husband when she had a clear reason for doing so and would resist the urge to call when worried about his safety.

Often clients identify more than one type of worry safety behavior. For example, a client might check her work repeatedly during the day, leave early for scheduled medical appointments, and call others for reassurance about social or relationship concerns. In these cases, therapists ask clients to select the worry safety behavior they expect would be easiest to give up. Response prevention assignments begin with this behavior first, advance to the second easiest behavior after the first has been mastered, and so on. Alternatively, various safety behaviors can be incorporated into a single hierarchy with specific tasks at increasing levels of difficulty. In the example above, the client might agree to leave on time (instead of early) for an upcoming medical appointment scheduled over the next week. Next, the client might select a particular low-priority work task in which she will forego any checking. Subsequent assignments might include leaving on time for a more important appointment, checking important documents at work only once, and refraining from asking for reassurance during conversations with friends. Clients continue to practice new response prevention assignments until they no longer engage in problematic worry safety behavior.

Naturally, most clients will express some hesitation when first presented with response prevention assignments. Therapists should prepare clients to expect anxiety before, as well as during, these assignments. Increased discomfort can be reframed as evidence that an appropriate response prevention task was selected. Clients expressing reluctance to try these assignments might benefit from discussion of what they fear could happen. These predictions can be examined with cognitive therapy procedures described in Chap. 6. Faulty causal attributions about worry safety behavior can be examined in the same fashion as described for positive worry beliefs. Successful relaxation home practice sessions provide good examples of times when clients did not engage in worry safety behavior. Clients might look to recent relaxation practice for evidence of what happens in the absence of worry behavior.

Clients might conduct behavioral experiments by refraining from the safety behavior for a limited time. Immediately afterward, clients compare what they feared would happen to what actually happened. Along similar lines, Rachman (2004) suggested a safety behavior "off-duty" period. Clients select an hour each day and spend that time free from planning or any other preventive behavior, much like an air-traffic controller does not need to scan the flight screen while off duty. Borkovec and colleagues (2004) described a variation on the worry postponement procedure involving "worry-free zones." Worry is put off during a certain time, place, or activity each day. This worry-free zone gradually expands to include more times, places, and activities over the course of treatment. For many clients, formal relaxation practice sessions serve the dual purpose of relaxation skill development and respite from safety behavior and worry. Thus, reluctant clients could begin their response prevention efforts with a limited off-duty, worry-free zone in addition to ongoing relaxation practice sessions. Each week therapists review client progress and compare feared outcomes to actual outcomes. Clients expand their off-duty/worry-free zones until response prevention of all worry safety behaviors has occurred.

Cost-benefit analysis provides a final option for clients hesitant to try response prevention assignments. Therapists explain that most people perform adaptive safety behaviors on a routine basis, such as wearing a seatbelt. In this example, however, the cost is low and the potential benefit is high: buckling the seatbelt takes only a moment, and the increased protection provided in the event of a car accident is significant. In contrast, worry safety behaviors cost unnecessary time and effort and maintain anxious disturbance. Immediate short-term relief is typically the only true benefit to these behaviors, as any perceived protective benefits are minimal at best. Clients become willing to try initial response prevention assignments as they realize the true cost of worry safety behavior. The advantage of achieving stated therapy goals outweighs the small advantage of short-term relief from temporary distress.

## Passive Avoidance Behavior

Clinicians most often associate the anxiety disorders with this second type of avoidance behavior. Passive avoidance involves escape from feared activities, situations, or stimuli, as well as a failure to approach them in the first place. Many clients with GAD do avoid specific objects or situations associated with common phobias. However, much of the passive avoidance behavior seen in GAD can be quite subtle and difficult to identify. Furthermore, such avoidance behavior does not always cause obvious distress or impairment. Clients may not even be aware that they avoid certain stimuli, activities, or situations connected to their worry. In contrast to other anxiety disorders, the DSM-IV GAD diagnostic criteria do not include behavioral avoidance. Nevertheless, passive avoidance behavior can prevent crucial learning experiences for clients, thereby maintaining threat interpretations and undermining treatment efforts. Once specific avoided situations are identified, clients rank order each and place on an exposure hierarchy. Clients conduct *in vivo* exposure assignments between sessions, starting with low-ranking items and gradually working their way up the hierarchy.

## *Identifying Passive Avoidance Behavior*

Many clients with GAD fear and avoid circumscribed objects or situations. The initial diagnostic assessment typically reveals any specific phobias that might be present, such as fear of air travel, heights, elevators, or certain animals. Therapists ask clients to list any situation they avoid out of concern for their physical safety. In addition to easily identified phobic stimuli, physical safety worries may reveal more subtle avoidance behavior. For example, a client who worries about car accidents might avoid driving only to an extent. This client may drive to any destination she needs, but routinely selects surface street routes to avoid the freeway and always avoids heavy traffic areas. Thus, passive avoidance behavior may not present at the severity required for comorbid specific phobia diagnosis. Clients worried about physical safety also might avoid simple daily activities, such as reading, watching, or listening to the news. These clients may habitually change the television channel or radio station whenever a news report appears. Similarly, clients may change the topic whenever a tragic event comes up in the course of a conversation. Clients also may avoid travel due to perceptions of increased risk while away from home. Overprotective parenting behavior may include both active and passive avoidance behaviors, including refusal to hire a babysitter or not permitting children to stay alone with trusted family members or friends.

During discussions of avoided situations, therapists readily acknowledge that clients must assume some level of risk with any activity. No guarantees of complete safety can be made. Risks are only relative in nature, with some risks considered not worth taking and other risks too small to warrant behavioral avoidance. Just as some safety behaviors might be considered adaptive (e.g., wearing a seatbelt while driving, wearing a helmet when riding a bicycle), passive avoidance of high risk situations is also functional. However, avoidance behavior based upon inflated perception of risk is overly conservative and therefore will perpetuate unnecessary anxiety and impose excessive limits on client experiences. As avoided activities or situations are identified, therapists help clients determine whether avoidance of each is truly adaptive versus worth changing with gradual exposure assignments.

Many perceived threats found among individuals with GAD are social in nature. Among individuals diagnosed with GAD, social phobia is the most frequently diagnosed comorbid condition (Brown & Barlow 1992). Social and interpersonal concerns comprise the most frequently reported worry topic, regardless of diagnostic status (e.g., Roemer, Molina, & Borkovec 1997). Thus, clients may avoid various social situations and interactions, such as asserting themselves or saying "no," approaching people in authority positions, striking up conversations, dating, or public speaking situations. Clients without signs of social phobia still might avoid intimate interpersonal interactions in which they feel vulnerable to rejection. For example, some clients might enjoy socializing at parties yet avoid disclosing personal information and expressing genuine emotion to loved ones or close friends.

In addition to passive avoidance of intimate interactions, such clients might engage in active avoidance behaviors also designed to prevent rejection. Pincus and Borkovec (1994) found that clients with GAD reported problematic interpersonal behavior characterized as "overly nurturant and intrusive" more often than non anxious participants. We not only replicated this result, but also found that individuals with GAD reported this particular interpersonal behavior pattern more than a panic disorder comparison group (Shoenberger & Hazlett-Stevens in press). Such interpersonal difficulties were negatively associated with clinical improvement following CBT treatment (Borkovec, Newman, Pincus, & Lytle 2002). Thus, clients may have adopted overbearing forms of caretaking behavior which not only maintain anxiety, but inadvertently cause the very same negative interpersonal consequences clients fear. As described previously, Newman and colleagues have extended traditional CBT to target both active and passive forms of interpersonal avoidance behavior found in GAD (Newman, Castonguay, Borkovec, & Molnar 2004).

Passive avoidance behavior also stems from fears of failure or incompetence and subsequent worry about task performance. Procrastination, the classic form of work-related passive avoidance behavior, involves unnecessarily postponing work. Clients avoid working on important tasks due to fears that the end product will not meet expected standards. Clients also might fear that tasks will not get completed on time; ironically, this very possibility increases as procrastination continues. While procrastinating, clients might fill their time with distracting activity such as housecleaning, watching television, playing video games, or surfing the internet. Procrastination can be addressed with the same exposure therapy method developed for other types of passive avoidance behavior. First, full-scale projects are broken down into a series of specific concrete tasks. Each task then becomes an exposure assignment, with more manageable preparatory work tasks placed near the bottom of the exposure hierarchy. Clients plan ahead of time exactly where, when, and for how long they will work on the selected task. For projects on a tight timeline, clients might decide to complete an exposure assignment each day. Clients are encouraged to focus only on the assigned task at hand, as contemplating the entire project at once soon becomes overwhelming.

## Eliminating Passive Avoidance Behavior with Exposure Assignments

After clients have identified any specific activities, situations, and stimuli avoided, therapists help them construct a systematic plan for exposure. Clients start with manageable exposure assignments to gain mastery over feared situations. In subsequent assignments, therapists and clients select activities expected to produce optimal levels of anxiety. That is, each assigned exposure activity ideally produces a moderate amount of anxiety that is neither too low nor overwhelmingly high. This gradual approach is accomplished by creating an exposure hierarchy. Therapists and clients work together to create a list of situations for exposure. Clients rate each situation for its expected anxiety using the 0–100 rating scale introduced at the beginning of treatment. Feared situations are then rank ordered from lowest to highest, and each week a new exposure assignment is selected. Clients begin with low hierarchy items and work their way up to the most difficult situations.

In cases of GAD, therapists often have difficulty creating a single hierarchy because clients typically fear an array of activities or situations. Generating items for a hierarchy is more straightforward when only a single situation is feared. Thus, one approach is to tackle one situation at a time, with hierarchy items representing increasingly difficult tasks related to the selected feared situation. For example, a client with multiple safety-related fears and worries might start with exposure exercises targeting driving avoidance behavior. Lower hierarchy items might involve listening to the traffic report on the radio while driving a usual "safe" route. Later exposure assignments might involve a brief trip on the freeway spanning the length of one freeway exit. Eventually, exposure assignments at the top of the hierarchy would involve driving long distances on unfamiliar stretches of road without another person in the car or other objects perceived to increase safety. Once all driving avoidance behavior has been addressed, fear of flying could be addressed with a new set of gradual hierarchy items.

A second approach might be to group similar situations together into a couple of different hierarchies and assign one exposure exercise from each on a weekly basis. For example, a client may have multiple social fears as well as several idiosyncratic physical safety avoidance behaviors. Her social situation hierarchy may involve approaching a co-worker for help near the bottom and asking upper-level management for a raise near the top. A separate physical safety hierarchy might involve items such as watching 10 min of national news each evening, followed by leaving a child with a trusted babysitter for an evening out. In addition to conducting formal exposure assignments between sessions, clients are encouraged to stay in feared situations rather than give in to escape urges whenever feasible.

Once the therapist and client have agreed upon a specific hierarchy item for the upcoming week, the client details a specific plan for exposure. When and where does he or she plan to approach the previously avoided activity? What exactly does he or she plan to do? Therapists provide the following instructions to maximize the likelihood of effective self-directed exposure assignments:

1. Approach the situation directly, exactly as planned. As you enter the situation or begin the activity, experience both your surroundings and your own internal reactions as fully as you can. Your natural anxiety response should be welcomed rather than resisted. Instead of "white-knuckling" through the exposure, behave as if you were not afraid. Take your time with the task, noticing what really happens as well as how you feel. Stay in the situation as long as you can—either until the activity comes to an end or until you notice your anxiety has run its course and naturally declines.

2. Rate your anxiety immediately before and immediately after each exposure attempt. Keep track of these anxiety levels as you repeat the exposure assignment.

3. After your first practice attempt, repeat the exposure again. Keep repeating the exposure assignment until it produces only mild anxiety.

4. If you notice your anxiety does not reduce with exposure, ask yourself why this might be happening. Are you rehearsing threatening interpretations of the situation

instead of tuning into what is happening around you? In this case, try an easier version of the exercise you think would be more manageable.

5. If you do not feel much anxiety during exposure, also ask yourself why this might be happening. Are you doing something to feel "safe" instead of allowing yourself to experience fear? Are you carrying a safety object to feel more comfortable? Try the exposure exercise again without any safety behavior and see what happens.

In each subsequent session, the therapist discusses the client's experience with exposure assignments. Previous assignments can be revised or repeated for the next week if difficulties were reported. Therapists guide clients to problem-solve any practical obstacles to successful practice. Therapists consistently encourage client efforts, reminding clients that progress is not always steady and upward. Minor setbacks can be reframed as challenges to be expected instead of evidence that clients cannot benefit from exposure. In addition to structured exposure exercises, therapists encourage other forms of flexible behavior. Clients might experiment with trying new or unfamiliar activities. Many simple changes to routine, such as eating at a new restaurant, making a new dinner recipe, or shopping in an unfamiliar store, challenge established habits, thereby promoting more purposeful and flexible behavior.

## Imagery Exposure and Coping Rehearsal

Over the past 25 years, a variety of imagery exposure techniques have been developed to treat GAD. Early theory conceptualized worry a means to avoid catastrophic images (Borkovec 1994), based on research demonstrating a predominance of verbal thought activity over visual imagery during worry. Borkovec and Inz (1990) asked individuals with GAD and a nonanxious comparison group to engage in both worry and self-relaxation in the laboratory. Each participant was briefly interrupted throughout each period to report whether that current thought was comprised of verbal thought versus imagery. Participants with GAD reported equivalent amounts of verbal thought and imagery during relaxation, whereas the nonanxious group reported significantly more imagery than verbal thought. During worry, both participant groups reported a predominance of verbal thought. A later investigation replicated these effects and found that the number of somatic symptoms endorsed was positively correlated with the percentage of images reported (Freeston, Dugas, & Ladouceur 1996). Among excessive worriers, the number of autonomic hyperactivity symptoms was negatively correlated with the percentage of verbal thoughts. In a final series of investigations, non-worry topics involved more imagery than worry topics, increased worry about a given topic was associated with less imagery, and imagery that did occur during worry appeared not to be very concrete (Stöber 1998; Stöber, Tepperwien, & Staak 2000). Why might individuals with GAD be motivated to avoid worry-related visual imagery more so than covertly talking to themselves about the worry topic? Imagery elicits greater physiological emotional response than verbal articulation of the same event (Vrana, Cuthbert, & Lang 1986). Thus, clients with GAD might engage in worry to avoid even more intense negative affect from visual images. Imagery exposure techniques therefore target the feared images clients theoretically avoid with worry.

In one imagery exposure approach (Zinbarg, Craske, & Barlow 2006; Craske & Barlow 2006a), truly catastrophic images are selected for exposure. Clients repeatedly imagine vivid scenes representing worst possible outcomes. Often these images involve tragic or violent events, such as serious physical injury or death of a loved one. Consistent with the behavior therapy principles underlying desensitization, clients habituate to distressing images with repeated prolonged exposure. Eventually clients generate vivid and concrete images of feared catastrophic events without evoking a strong emotional response. However, feared catastrophic images among individuals with GAD differ from feared imagery associated with other anxiety disorders in potentially important ways. Unlike images of phobic stimuli, typical GAD imagery does not reflect present reality; the feared scenario does not actually exist in the present moment. Furthermore, the phobic stimuli captured in phobia-related imagery are not inherently harmful whereas worry-related catastrophic images may represent instances of true physical harm. In contrast to imagery selected for exposure among trauma survivors, the feared images associated with GAD represent only hypothetical events rather than past events that indeed already have occurred. Given the illusory nature of GAD-related feared images, concerns about possible counter-therapeutic effects of this imagery exposure approach could be raised. Images of events might be stored similar to memories for actual past events, as imagined fictional events can be recalled as having actually happened (Garry, Manning, & Loftus 1996). Catastrophic imagery exposure therefore might further inflate perceived probabilities of unlikely future tragedies, undermining cognitive therapy efforts. For this reason, exposure to images of truly catastrophic yet unreal events may be contraindicated in the treatment of GAD.

A second approach to worry-related imagery exposure involves likely scenarios in which ultimate outcomes are somewhat ambiguous. Clients might imagine feared upcoming employment situations or anticipated social interactions. During imagery exposure, clients allow and experience emotional arousal while visualizing adaptive coping as subsequent events unfold. Clients are encouraged to imagine probable and realistic outcomes during this scene rather than highly unlikely outcomes considered either ideal or catastrophic. The purpose of this imagery exposure method is twofold. The first goal is the same as described above: clients face upcoming feared situations in imagery to allow for extinction of anxious responding. Second, this imagery technique provides a means for rehearsing adaptive coping behavior in the context of relevant situations.

This imagery exposure method, self-control desensitization, was first developed by Goldfried (1971) for diffuse anxiety clinical presentations. Borkovec and colleagues later adapted the original Goldfried therapy procedure as a component of their CBT treatment package for GAD (Borkovec et al. 2002). Clients identify specific situations expected to generate anxiety. Next, clients close their eyes and enter a relaxed state. When relaxed, clients imagine themselves in the feared situation with any associated anxiety spiral cues. Clients notice and allow initial anxiety responses then deploy applied relaxation and cognitive coping skills. Clients continue to imagine themselves coping with the situation until directed to stop. This procedure is repeated for each situation until imagery exposure no longer elicits an initial anxiety response. These self-control desensitization procedures developed by Borkovec and colleagues at the Penn State GAD project are described next.

## Selecting Imagery Exposure Scenes

Therapists might review the rationale for imagery exposure presented near the beginning of treatment. Through imagery, clients gain additional practice identifying anxiety cues and reacting with coping responses. Rather than wait for actual worrisome situations to arrive, clients can practice implementing coping responses beforehand using their imagination. Repeated live exposure teaches clients to experience actual situations in a new way; likewise, repeated exposure to images representing future feared situations eventually makes these situations less anxiety-provoking.

Therapists and clients next generate a list of scenarios clients could practice in imagery. Clients might select a current worry topic, then describe a specific feared situation reflecting that worry. Each imagery exposure scene should contain an isolated incident that can be vividly imagined with concrete details. Selected scenes could represent actual upcoming events clients fear, such as an annual job evaluation feedback session or a scheduled public speaking appearance. Imagery exposure scenes also might represent *in vivo* exposure assignments clients prefer to practice in imagery first. Clients who cannot anticipate specific upcoming events might describe a likely hypothetical situation captured in their worry. In one example, a client worried about appearing foolish in the course of a conversation might not have any such conversations planned. However, he could construct a scenario in which he is talking to a particular person in a certain setting and cannot think of anything to say. Therapists can help clients generate a variety of possible situations, drawing from clinical information collected during assessment and previous cognitive therapy sessions.

Once clients have an array of possible scenarios, they rank order this list according to anxiety level. Their list should contain situations expected to elicit low, moderate, and high levels of anxiety and should cover each main worry topic. Just as described for live exposure procedures, clients ascend up a hierarchy in a graduated fashion. Clients first attempt imagery exposure in session with a low-anxiety scene. Clients might continue this imagery exposure practice at home between sessions, and then move on to the next hierarchy scenario in the following session. Clients should experience mastery with the procedure during mild anxiety situations before more distressing images are attempted. Before imagery exposure is conducted for each scene, therapists should ascertain several details about the scene and likely client responses. Exactly where will the scene take place, what other people will be present, and what are they likely to say and do? What anxiety spiral cues does the client anticipate, such as muscle tension, automatic anxious thoughts, or other bodily sensations? Therapists proceed with imagery exposure only after obtaining a clear picture of what the feared scene entails.

## *Conducting Imagery Exposure*

When clients are ready to begin the imagery exposure exercise, therapists ask them to sit back, close their eyes, and achieve a state of relaxation. Any of the relaxation procedures described in Chap. 5 may be used for this purpose. Therapists assist clients as much as needed to achieve deep relaxation, depending on the client's relaxation skills. Therapists also might add this procedure to the end of formal progressive relaxation practice. Once clients are relaxed, therapists remind them of the scene and instruct them to turn on the image. Clients visualize the scene while noticing anxiety cues and sensations as they occur. Clients should experience the scene as fully as they can, as if they were participating in the event at that moment. As clients imagine the scene, therapists describe aspects of the situation itself as well as anticipated client anxiety reactions. For example, a therapist guiding a client through imagery of a meeting with a work supervisor might say, "imagine yourself sitting in the chair across from your supervisor's desk…you notice a serious look on his face and feel your muscles tense up."

Clients are instructed to signal to the therapist, by lifting their hand or a finger, as soon as they notice a shift away from relaxation. When clients make this gesture, therapists instruct them to stay in the scene and experience the anxiety. After approximately 1 min, therapists instruct clients to imagine they are coping in the scene. Clients imagine themselves letting go of anxiety cues, deploying relaxation responses, and covertly saying alternative coping statements. Therapists guide clients through coping imagery as well with statements such as "imagine yourself taking a deep breath, reminding yourself you can cope with this situation." Clients continue this coping imagery until they signal to therapists that the anxiety has passed. Clients continue to imagine themselves in the scene calm and relaxed for another 20–30 seconds. Lastly, clients are instructed to turn off the image and enjoy relaxation for a final 20–30 seconds. This full procedure is immediately repeated three times or until clients no longer signal anxiety after turning on the imagery scene.

Once clients have finished the imagery exposure exercise and opened their eyes, therapists ask about their experience. Were they able to get a clear and vivid image? Were they able to experience themselves coping in the situation? Clients reporting some difficulty might benefit from repeating this procedure with the same image. Alternatively, clients who did not experience anxiety might select a more anxiety-provoking image. Clients who found the image more distressing than expected might repeat the procedure with a less anxiety-provoking version of the scenario.

Therapists encourage clients to try this imagery exposure exercise at home, repeating the exposure procedure until the image no longer generates much anxiety. In subsequent sessions, therapists guide clients through the procedure with a new scene of greater difficulty. Clients continue to identify specific upcoming events for future imagery exposure practice. Furthermore, as clients notice any distressing imagery in the course of daily life, they can practice envisioning themselves coping with probable outcomes.

## Lifestyle Behavior Change

The behavior therapy procedures described above target active and passive avoidance behaviors believed to maintain perceptions of threat and anxious disturbance. Indeed, systematic confrontation of feared situations and activities may be crucial to therapy success. However, many clients also neglect desired activities and behaviors when preoccupied with avoiding feared outcomes. When a client's primary motivation is to minimize threat, many life choices are made from this perspective. Goals to live a full and enriched life give way to objectives such as achieving certainty or preventing as many dangers as possible. Leisure activities and health-promoting behaviors are difficult to initiate while overwhelmed with symptoms of anxiety and depression. Clients suffering from GAD often describe living a life of deprivation, void of pleasure, excitement, or joy.

As clients achieve initial cognitive and behavior change, they may benefit from a large-scale examination of their current lifestyle. Additional therapy goals beyond symptom improvement are identified, such as increasing meaningful and rewarding activities that are important to clients yet have been overlooked or neglected. Clients might discover that career or educational pursuits have been hindered by fears of failure. Healthy diet and regular exercise habits may have been neglected or perhaps were never established. Clients are encouraged to examine their life priorities beyond anxiety-driven aims of detecting threat and avoiding negative consequences. Clients identify which life activities they value most as well as any enjoyable activities they wish they did more often. Similar behavior therapies originally developed for depression, such as scheduling pleasant events (e.g., Lewinsohn 1975) and behavioral activation (e.g., Martell 2003), were based on the principle that engagement in desired activities increases positive reinforcement from the environment. Client efforts previously invested in threat detection can be redirected into personally meaningful and rewarding pursuits.

### *Identifying Neglected Activities*

Therapists might begin with pointed questions such as how clients would spend their time if they were suddenly free from worry and anxiety. In the course of discussion, GAD can be reframed as an opportunity for clients to take an inventory of their life choices. What matters most to them besides anticipating and preventing threat? Clients are encouraged to take a good look at their lifestyle behavior, career decisions, and ways in which they currently spend their time. How does current reality compare to clients' stated personal values? Often clients realize they have neglected their physical health, spent little quality time with loved ones, or abandoned favorite pastimes involving art, music, or nature. For example, some clients might claim to prioritize spending time with their children, yet work 70-hour weeks consistently without taking vacations. Other clients might discover that they chose a line of work that seemed predictable and familiar over more rewarding career paths they envisioned during their college years.

Such discussions may elicit strong emotion. Clients might be surprised by their own emotional reactions, as discovering large discrepancies between stated values and current life situations can be quite upsetting at first. Clients also may express feeling defeated, believing that they must live according to past choices and are stuck in their current circumstances indefinitely. Therapists respond with genuine empathy and support while emphasizing the crucial role of conscious choice. Therapists help clients appreciate they have behavioral options and are capable of taking action. Although clients occasionally decide to make dramatic life changes, such as starting a new career or relocating to a new part of the country, most clients can incorporate simple behavior changes to live more in accord with their true desires and values.

## Increasing Engagement in Desired Activities

Once clients have identified specific neglected activities, they can generate a detailed plan for change. Similar to behavior exposure exercises, clients might decide to start small. For example, clients might commit to engage in one previously neglected leisure activity over the first week. Assigned activities could be as simple as listening to a favorite piece of music for a short time. Clients also might commit to certain behaviors needed to pave the way for increased desired activity. For example, a client without any leisure time due to a heavy workload might commit to specific steps needed to take some time off work. Clients might benefit further from written assignments such as exploring life priorities in a journal or compiling a list of leisure activities they wish to pursue.

As clients engage in each activity, they should try to immerse themselves in that activity as much as possible. Clients are encouraged to focus their attention on the present moment as much as possible, making each action purposeful and deliberate. As practiced during formal relaxation sessions, clients bring their mind back to the present moment whenever they notice it has wandered. Clients familiar with the concept of mindfulness can approach each desired activity assignment as an opportunity for mindfulness practice. As Borkovec (2002) suggested, clients can increase their enjoyment of activities significantly when they focus on process over outcome. As clients experience the process involved with a given activity, they become less preoccupied with possible outcomes or results. Clients are encouraged to approach other activities and tasks in this manner, such as work assignments or household chores. Borkovec further recommended that clients identify intrinsic sources of motivation for such routine activities. Rather than perform tasks for the sole purpose of producing external consequences, clients can explore why else they might have chosen the activity. For example, a client may be motivated to write an article for extrinsic reasons such as maintaining satisfactory job performance and earning a salary. However, she might have chosen a career that involves writing articles because writing offers her intrinsic rewards of discovering new information and developing original ideas. The longer she writes while connected to her intrinsic motivation, the more enjoyment she likely will gain from her work. Conversely, the longer she writes while focused on external motivators, the greater the potential for disappointment and other negative affect. Ironically, focus on intrinsic reward ultimately may improve work quality and therefore increase the likelihood of external reward as well.

## Chapter Summary

Despite the free-floating and diffuse nature of anxiety associated with GAD, many clients exhibit a wide array of subtle avoidance behavior. Active avoidance is characterized by various worry safety behaviors. Clients engage in acts such as excessive checking or repeated reassurance-seeking to feel secure or to prevent unwanted outcomes. Passive avoidance of circumscribed phobic situations as well as various social interactions also may be present. Avoidance of simple everyday activities is also common. For example, many clients with GAD avoid listening, watching, or reading the news or discussing worry-related topics in the course of conversation. Therapists and clients identify any instances of avoidance behavior that reinforce client perceptions of threat, thereby maintaining anxious meanings of feared events. Worry safety behaviors are gradually eliminated through response prevention assignments. Therapists target passive avoidance behavior by constructing an exposure hierarchy and assigning self-directed *in vivo* exposure practice.

Therapists conduct in-session exposure using a coping imagery rehearsal technique known as self-control desensitization. Clients generate a list of worry-related situations and arrange them into an imagery exposure hierarchy. Clients first achieve a state of relaxation, and then visualize a selected scene in vivid detail. Once clients experience initial anxiety, they practice responding to the scene with relaxation responses and coping self-statements. Imagery exposure scenes are repeated within a single practice session until imagining the scene no longer generates anxiety. Clients might practice imagery exposure at home before more difficult scenes are attempted in subsequent therapy sessions. Whenever clients notice distressing worry-related imagery, they can apply this coping imagery technique immediately. Rather than avoiding the distressing image altogether, clients instead imagine they are coping with probable outcomes.

In addition to feared situations and images, clients with GAD also tend to avoid activities that provide enjoyment and promote physical health. Artistic pursuits, exercise, hobbies, and spending leisure time with family, friends, and loved ones are easily neglected in the service of anticipating and preventing harm. Therapists raise this possibility with clients and encourage them to examine larger life priorities. In a systematic fashion, clients return to neglected desired activities and make other life changes in accord with their true personal values and priorities.

# Chapter 8
# Common Problems and Clinical Considerations

Over the course of therapy, a variety of pitfalls may occur. Problems in treatment most often are revealed when clients express reluctance toward home practice assignments or fail to complete them between sessions. Poor homework compliance can arise from factors ranging from a breakdown in the therapeutic alliance to practical time management difficulties. Other complications are associated with specific treatment components. For example, relaxation techniques occasionally produce paradoxical increases in anxiety. During cognitive therapy, clients may experience difficulty performing initial thought tracking steps or responding to Socratic questions. In some cases, clients may misapply cognitive therapy techniques such that substituting new thoughts functions as a new covert worry safety behavior. Behavior therapy and live exposure exercises do not always go as planned, and some clients have difficulty engaging in imagery exposure. A final clinical consideration arises as therapy termination approaches: relapse prevention. Therapists prepare clients for continued practice of new skills after therapy sessions have ended to ensure that therapy gains persist. Therapists and clients outline a detailed plan of action designed to maintain therapy gains and guide client responses to future challenges and return of symptoms. Clients leave their final session with this structured written relapse prevention plan in place.

## Poor Compliance with Home Assignments

Failure to follow through with assigned home exercises typically appears early in treatment. Clients may have difficulty with initial self-monitoring or they may be ambivalent about making the commitment required for effective CBT. Nevertheless, the general difficulties described below also apply to subsequent home practice assignments involving relaxation, cognitive therapy, behavior therapy, and exposure techniques. Sometimes these complications do not arise until later in treatment. Some clients immerse themselves in treatment initially then become disillusioned when dramatic improvements are not immediate. Certainly most clients fail to complete home assignments on occasion, and these instances may provide useful information about client perceptions. When problems with homework compliance

H. Hazlett-Stevens, *Psychological Approaches to Generalized Anxiety Disorder*,
doi: 10.1007/978-0-387-76870-0, © Springer Science+Business Media, LLC 2008

persist, the common reasons described below can serve as a checklist for clinicians. For additional information and clinical suggestions regarding homework compliance the reader is referred to Waters and Craske (2005) and Leahy (2005b).

## Low Motivation to Participate in Treatment

Clients easily become overwhelmed when therapists ask them to devote time each day to home assignments. Clients often claim they are already overcommitted and do not have any more time to spend on therapy exercises between sessions. Rather than apologize for the effort therapy requires, therapists can empathize with any client ambivalence. Therapists might encourage clients to describe any potential benefits or eventual "payoffs" that might be worth the required time and energy. During this discussion, therapists also review any information contained in the CBT rationale that may not have been explained clearly or that clients may not have understood fully. Newman (2000) recommended that therapists ask clients to view the time spent with homework assignments as an investment. Lowering unnecessary anxiety "costs" extensive time and effort up front. However, this investment eventually saves time. Clients typically function better and therefore accomplish more with successful treatment. In their discussion of panic disorder treatment obstacles, McCabe and Antony (2005) recommended that therapists address low motivation directly with motivation enhancement techniques (Miller & Rollnick 2002). These interventions, such as identifying discrepancies between client goals and problem behaviors, emphasizing personal control, and drawing client attention to personal strengths, also may help clients with GAD contemplating change.

Finally, clients ambivalent about therapy might "argue" each side of their ambivalence using the two-chair technique described in Chap. 6. While sitting in one chair, the client voices all the benefits and reasons they want to engage in therapy and to change. Therapists periodically ask clients to switch to the opposing chair and argue back, describing all of the drawbacks, fears, and reasons for their reluctance. Often this exercise will reveal underlying beliefs that could hinder progress in therapy. For example, strong positive worry beliefs that worry reduction will somehow make clients more vulnerable to harm could be identified and addressed. These meta-cognitive beliefs could be examined near the beginning of treatment with the cognitive therapy techniques described in Chap. 6. Therapists also might discover that a significant other person has contributed to low client motivation. Clients may have adopted the skepticism or doubt expressed by close friends and family members, particularly others who stand to benefit from the client's anxiety and avoidant behavior. Clients themselves may identify subtle gains associated with their current condition, such as evading certain responsibilities or receiving sympathy from others. As therapists engage clients in a frank discussion of the pros and cons, clients are encouraged to arrive at their own decision about whether or not they are willing to make a commitment to CBT and behavior change.

## *Practical Problems Completing Home Assignments*

Some clients may be quite motivated to change, yet have significant difficulty organizing activities and managing their time. Such clients often report they forgot to follow through with home assignments when the time came. Other difficulties include getting absorbed in a task and losing track of time, thereby working through the time period selected for home practice. Therapists reframe these practical difficulties as problems to be solved and then help clients generate solutions to try over the next week. For example, Newman (2000) suggested that clients who forget to do home assignments identify ways to remind themselves within their daily environment. Post-it notes could be placed on objects such as the telephone, computer, or daily calendar. Frequent reminders to engage in self-monitoring from the external environment eventually lead to new habits and internal prompts.

Clients with severe time management difficulties may overextend themselves regularly, underestimating the time required for each activity. Perfectionist tendencies may complicate matters further if clients spend significantly more time than needed to accomplish routine tasks. As a result, home practice assignments quickly become neglected. Once clients have prioritized therapy home practice assignments, these problems can be addressed directly with time management strategies. Craske and Barlow (2006a) outlined four specific steps clients can take to manage their time more efficiently: delegating responsibility, saying "no," sticking to an agenda, and avoiding perfectionism. Clients begin to incorporate these four steps into their daily lives by tracking intended and accomplished activities on a "Daily Activities" form. Therapy-related tasks and home practice assignments are included on this form as planned activities with high priority. Leahy (2004) reported that clients with GAD who struggle with perfectionism often benefit from reading Monica Basco's *Never Good Enough* (2000). In addition to improving homework compliance, time management interventions teach clients to work more effectively in many areas of their life. Clients increasingly become more able to take on future therapy assignments, including enjoyable leisure activities.

## *Fear that Homework Will Increase Anxiety and Worry*

Sometimes clients report that although they want to address their anxiety in therapy, they also fear that talking, thinking, and writing about anxious material will only make them worse. Therapists can acknowledge the natural desire to avoid activities that cause discomfort while emphasizing the benefits of the new approach offered in treatment. Therapists might help clients examine beliefs that they could not tolerate temporary distress or periodic increases in anxiety. In addition, homework assignments differ from usual worry in important ways. The belief that all home assignments will in fact lead to increased anxiety can be tested with behavioral experiments. Failure to complete home assignments can be conceptualized as another form of behavioral avoidance. Putting off a homework task may effectively decrease anxiety in the short term, but this choice only perpetuates anxious disturbance in the long run. Therapists might engage clients in a cost-benefit analysis in which accepting the risk of feeling more anxious may yield future benefits such as symptom reduction or improved functioning. As discussed in Chap. 6, clients who often engage in meta-worry (i.e., worry about worry) hold beliefs that any additional anxiety or worry will lead them to go crazy or do something out of control. Once identified, these beliefs can be examined and restructured as described in Chap. 6. The reader also is referred to Wells (2000) for additional clinical suggestions regarding meta-worry.

## Problems in the Therapeutic Relationship

Another possible explanation for poor homework compliance is a strained therapeutic alliance. When a client perceives the therapist as uncaring or a client harbors negative feelings toward the therapist, a productive collaboration is no longer possible. Indeed, some clients may come to therapy with rigid and dysfunctional interpersonal styles that preclude establishment of a strong working alliance. For these clients, interpersonally-oriented interventions such as those described by Safran and Segal (1990) and by Kohlenberg and Tsai (Functional Analytic Psychotherapy; 1991) may be needed before proceeding with standard CBT. As described previously, Newman and colleagues (2004) recently developed an integrative treatment for GAD that incorporates many interpersonal therapy practices from Safran and Segal (1990).

In most cases, however, careful and sensitive therapist attention to any ruptures in the therapeutic alliance can improve the therapeutic relationship significantly. Burns and Auerbach (1996) outlined a series of steps clinicians could follow when faced with an empathic failure in the course of cognitive-behavioral treatment. Using the "disarming technique," the therapist finds an aspect of truth in the client's concern, however unreasonable the overall claim may seem to the therapist. The therapist next puts him or herself into the client's perspective as fully as possible. Empathy is expressed both by paraphrasing the client's view and by acknowledging how the client probably feels. Finally, gentle probing questions to learn more about how the client thinks and feels are asked. Along similar lines, Safran and Muran (2000) recommended that therapists accept responsibility for their own contributions to problematic therapy interactions. The therapist even might invite the client to explore the therapist's contribution to the interaction at hand. While a full discussion of the therapeutic alliance is beyond the scope of this book, the reader is referred to Burns and Auerbach as well as Safran and Muran for further information and additional clinical suggestions.

## Common Problems Associated with Specific CBT Strategies

In addition to the general problems discussed above, other difficulties may arise when implementing the specific therapy strategies presented in the previous three chapters. Relaxation training sometimes presents therapists with technical problems, and occasionally clients respond to initial relaxation sensations with increased discomfort or anxiety. Difficulties implementing cognitive therapy strategies are not uncommon, as clients may struggle with identification and examination of their specific anxious thoughts. Common problems with response prevention and *in vivo* exposure exercises include clients feeling too overwhelmed by anxiety to stay in the situation, or conversely, not experiencing much distress when first confronting feared situations. All types of client responses to exposure exercises can be reframed as learning opportunities for both the therapist and client, including client failure to attempt the exposure exercise in the first place. Such unplanned outcomes simply guide the selection of future home exposure exercises. Finally, complications with imagery exposure include client difficulty generating a vivid and believable image.

## Relaxation Strategies

A variety of technical problems may arise during progressive relaxation training. Many slight variations from the protocol outlined in Chap. 5 are trivial and do not require correction. Therapists must exercise their own clinical judgment to determine whether or not a problem is likely to disrupt relaxation training. After initial practice sessions, clients sometimes report difficulty achieving complete muscle relaxation or trouble keeping their attention focused on their muscles. Therapists can simply reassure clients that such initial problems are to be expected and should improve with practice. Supplemental mindfulness practice exercises or the diaphragmatic breathing mental focus tasks described in Chap. 5 may improve clients' ability to sustain focused attention further. Other complications warrant immediate problem solving to set the stage for successful relaxation practice. For example, clients may have trouble producing noticeable tension in a certain muscle group. Therapists can ask the client to try alternative ways of tensing that muscle group. On the other hand, clients might report physical pain or muscle cramping during muscle tension. In these cases, clients are reminded only to produce enough tension to create a sensation that differs from relaxation; tensing each muscle group as much as possible is not necessary. Experimenting with alternative ways to produce tension often helps in this situation as well. As mentioned in Chap. 5, muscles in the lower legs and feet are prone to cramping and therefore should not be tensed for longer than four to five seconds at a time. For additional progressive relaxation trouble-shooting suggestions, the reader is referred to Bernstein, Borkovec, and Hazlett-Stevens (2000).

One particular relaxation training complication sometimes arises among clients struggling with anxiety and worry: relaxation-induced anxiety. Occasionally clients report a paradoxical increase in anxiety in response to initial relaxation-related sensations. New relaxation sensations foreign to the individual can result in subjective feelings of vulnerability and uneasiness. Relaxation naturally requires focused attention on bodily sensations. Thus, clients with a hypersensitivity to bodily sensations might interpret physical relaxation effects as threatening. Along similar lines, clients might be disturbed by the loss of vigilance and control associated with a state of relaxation. Oftentimes clients respond to therapist reassurance that some initial discomfort is common, especially given how unfamiliar a state of relaxation feels for individuals who live with chronic anxiety and tension. Clients are encouraged to continue relaxation practice to see if they indeed become accustomed to relaxation sensations and eventually look forward to relaxation practice. Therapists might pose this option as an experiment: "Sometimes clients will find that after a bit of practice they get used to feeling relaxed and even look forward to their next practice. We could look at your own personal experience as an experiment and see what happens for you. How would you feel about trying relaxation practice a few more times to see if any changes happen for you?"

Clients who do not respond to therapist reassurance after initial relaxation-induced anxiety probably will be reluctant to engage in relaxation practice again. These clients may benefit from further intervention targeting their fears of relaxation before additional practice is assigned. Clients may hold firm positive worry beliefs that they must actively engage in threat detection and worry at all times to prevent threat. Such beliefs can be subjected to cognitive restructuring as described in Chap. 6. Therapists can treat subsequent relaxation practice assignments as behavioral experiments. Clients engage in a brief relaxation exercise as part of their "off-duty, worry-free zone" (see Chap. 7). Occurrences during this practice serve as evidence in the subsequent examination of the original worry belief. Finally, relaxation exercises might be reframed as feared events to be subjected to behavioral exposure. Therapists and clients work together to generate a hierarchy of relaxation-related activities for clients to confront in a gradual fashion, as described in Chap. 7. For example, clients might begin with five 30-second periods of relaxing imagery, graduate to ten-minute long diaphragmatic breathing practice, next add a mental focus task to diaphragmatic breathing, then move on to progressive relaxation exercises.

## Cognitive Strategies

Clients may report difficulty at any of the cognitive therapy steps outlined in Chap. 6. From the outset, clients may exhibit trouble narrowing vague and abstract worries down to specific automatic anxious thoughts. Therapists must provide continuous reassurance and encouragement to clients, reminding them that this first step may seem simple yet requires repeated practice and self-inquiry. Therapists can help by asking pointed questions to elicit client responses that are as exact and concrete as possible. For example, if the client is worried about something in the future, exactly what does he or she fear will happen? After a sufficient period of time has elapsed, how could an outside observer factually conclude whether or not the event occurred? Clients who continue to experience difficulty with this first step may benefit from the structured exercise developed by Hazlett-Stevens (2005) reprinted in Chap. 6.

Once clients have successfully identified automatic anxious thoughts, they might have difficulty responding in the moment as instructed. While clients usually are able to remind themselves the thought is only a thought and not a fact, they may fail to experience cognitive distancing at first. These clients may benefit from expanded cognitive defusion techniques designed to teach clients how to separate themselves from the literal meaning reflected in thought content (Luoma & Hayes 2003). Cognitive defusion is one of the primary aims of Acceptance and Commitment Therapy (ACT; Hayes, Strosahl, & Wilson 1999), a multi-faceted contextual behavior therapy. In addition to mindfulness practice, Roemer and Orsillo (2005) have integrated some of the acceptance strategies from ACT into their acceptance-based behavior therapy for GAD.

Clients also may have trouble determining whether immediate constructive problem-solving action can be taken or whether the automatic anxious thought should be postponed to their worry period. Some clients might mistake this instruction as encouragement to engage in worry safety behavior or passive avoidance behavior. For example, a client catches herself worrying that her child will fall and hurt himself while watching him play on the playground. She then responds by ending the play session early rather than identifying the worry as unproductive and postponing to her worry period. Clients who experience difficulty distinguishing concrete problems worthy of constructive action from unproductive worry may benefit from supplemental problem-solving training interventions. Such interventions also are indicated for clients who have trouble orienting to real problems and taking constructive action. In their cognitive-behavioral treatment for GAD, Dugas and Robichaud (2007) outlined specific steps to help clients recognize solvable problems, orient to such problems, and then apply specific problem-solving skills. When clients do attempt to postpone their worry to a worry period, some may report trouble re-focusing their attention on the present moment and engaging in the task at hand. These clients may benefit from supplemental mindfulness practice, such as the self-help mindfulness exercises described in Hazlett-Stevens (2005). Mindfulness therapy procedures are described in detail by Kabat-Zinn (1990) and by Segal, Williams, and Teasdale (2002). As previously described, Roemer and Orsillo (2005) recently integrated mindfulness practice into their GAD treatment package.

Clients also may experience difficulty with the specific cognitive therapy techniques designed to challenge automatic anxious thoughts. When asked to generate alternative interpretations or predictions, many clients first report they are at a loss. Clients become so accustomed to accepting their automatic anxious thoughts, they often experience difficulty engaging in more flexible cognitive processes. In these cases, Newman (2000) suggested that clinicians have clients practice generating alternatives to neutral topics, such as listing advantages and disadvantages of a sunny day. Once clients gain initial success with neutral topics, therapists might ask them to generate alternatives their friends or family might generate if they were present. As discussed in Chap. 6, clients generating only negative alternatives can be encouraged to cover the full spectrum of possible outcomes from best to worst.

Two common problems arise while examining the evidence. The first reflects a classic client complaint encountered by most seasoned cognitive therapists: although the arguments against the automatic anxious thought make perfect logical sense and the client accepts each intellectually, the automatic anxious thought or underlying core belief still "feels true." This phenomenon is easily understood in cases of GAD. During the course of the worry process, clients experience intermittent intrusive catastrophic images. Although verbal-linguistic worry serves to avoid further unwanted imagery and associated affect (see Borkovec, Alcaine, & Behar 2004), periodic imagery, when it does occur, may inflate subjective probabilities of feared outcomes (Borkovec, Hazlett-Stevens, & Diaz 1999). Thus, clients feel as though unlikely events are quite likely to occur because such disasters often have occurred in their imagination. Some clients may respond to a discussion of this property of worry and imagery, as therapists offer a reasonable explanation for the observed discrepancy between what clients know intellectually and how they feel. Therapists and clients then could examine client expectations that automatic anxious thoughts suddenly will no longer "feel true" despite several years or even a lifetime of habitual cognitive activity.

Clients also may experience this phenomenon while restructuring underlying core beliefs, such as long-standing views that the self is incompetent or unworthy of others' love. In these cases, further exploration of these beliefs using experiential therapy techniques may be indicated. In their new Interpersonal/Emotional Processing (I/EP) therapy for GAD, Newman and colleagues (2004) employ simple emotional deepening interventions such as encouraging clients to stay with their emotions and pointing out when clients seem to move away from primary emotional experience in session. Emotions associated with negative core beliefs might be elicited with the two-chair exercise, in which clients speak from each side of the core belief or internal conflict separately as if each part of the self were two separate people. Alternatively, clients expressing unresolved feelings toward another person associated with the core belief may engage in the empty chair exercise described in Chap. 6 (Greenberg, Rice, & Elliott 1996).

Another complication arises when clients demand certainty or otherwise express an intolerance of uncertainty. During the course of examining the evidence, clients may insist that any degree of risk is intolerable or that worry cannot be suspended until they achieve complete certainty. This problem also arises while decatastrophizing, as the uncertain ramifications of any given situation are increasingly exposed. Therapists can engage clients in a discussion of the uncertainty inherent in life, challenging views that one can live in the world without accepting any level of risk or ambiguity. In their cognitive model of GAD, Dugas and Robichaud (2007) identified intolerance of uncertainty as a dispositional characteristic that places individuals at a heightened risk for GAD. Their treatment approach therefore targets this cognitive feature directly with interventions designed to identify client manifestations of intolerance of uncertainty and to expose clients to feared uncertainty-inducing situations. The reader is referred to Dugas and Robichaud for specific clinical suggestions aimed at reducing intolerance of uncertainty.

One final complication is associated with the application of coping self-statements. As presented in Chap. 6, clients end the cognitive therapy process by developing new perspectives and preventive beliefs. Clients apply these new perspectives in the form of coping self-statements, rehearsed as new responses to anxiety spiral cues. Clients sometimes misapply this strategy, merely substituting coping self-statements for automatic anxious thoughts to achieve immediate reassurance. This practice effectively transforms cognitive restructuring into a covert worry safety behavior, in which coping self-statements only increase perceptions of threat and prevent corrective learning experiences. If therapists suspect coping self-statements are serving an active avoidance function, they can raise this possibility with clients and look at their self-statements carefully. Superficial statements of reassurance, such as "Everything will be okay," lack essential properties. New perspectives should be balanced and flexible, reflecting the complexity and uncertainty of the situation. Once clients generate more appropriate coping self-statements, therapists also advise clients to return to the full thought tracking procedure before rehearsing the new perspective. Thus, clients work through each cognitive therapy step before coping self-statements are applied. A form of response prevention also is achieved when clients work through each cognitive therapy step rather than immediately engage in coping self-statements.

## *Behavior Therapy and Exposure Techniques*

Given the anxiety-provoking nature of response prevention and exposure exercises, clients understandably may report feeling overwhelmed by them. Clients either feel so overwhelmed with anticipatory anxiety they fail to attempt the exercise or they are unable to stay in the situation long enough for natural anxiety reduction to occur. The opposite may happen as well: some clients may engage in subtle safety behavior during exposure such that little anxiety is experienced. Whenever clients come to session and report problems with response prevention or exposure home assignments, therapists respond with support and encouragement. Each assignment outcome provides important feedback to the therapist and client, guiding plans for future assignments. Even failed attempts convey information about the strength of client fears, indicating the need to construct additional incremental steps on the hierarchy. If clients report the anxiety was too intense to conduct the assignment as planned, therapists work with them to create a new version that seems more manageable. Therapists also could invite clients to practice the assignment in imagery first before leaving the session.

   If clients did not experience much anxiety during the assignment, therapists invite clients to explore why this might have happened. Did the client inadvertently do something to feel safe, such as rehearsing empty self-reassurance statements or mental distraction? If so, a conscious effort to prevent this response during exposure is needed. Perhaps contextual details of the situation prevented the elicitation of anxiety or discomfort. In this case, therapists ask clients how the situation might differ so that immediate anxiety responses are provoked. Sometimes clients return to session pleasantly surprised by this "problem," having discovered that a situation they expected would overwhelm them actually was quite manageable. These clients sometimes choose to skip the next step on their hierarchy and attempt a more challenging assignment over the next week.

Other difficulties specific to imagery exposure procedures sometimes occur. During initial imagery attempts, clients may report that they cannot visualize a clear and vivid image. Many times therapist encouragement and reassurance that repeated practice helps build imagery skills are sufficient. Clients might continue with imagery relaxation practice for a while longer before attempting imagery exposure exercises again. After mastery with relaxing images, clients might practice imagining neutral scenes. Therapists ask clients to describe each imagery scene in great detail to ensure that only specific and concrete images are attempted. In a related complication, clients may find that imagining feared scenes do not generate much anxiety because imagery is not real. Therapists question clients about any features of the feared situation that might be missing. What might be added to the scenario that would help the client "get into" the image? Therapists then remind clients of the most salient internal and external anxiety cues during in-session therapist-guided imagery exposure.

## Therapy Termination and Relapse Prevention

As clients achieve therapy goals and demonstrate adaptive behavior change, therapists must determine when to initiate the termination process. Clients may raise the issue of termination themselves after they gain mastery over home assignments and successfully apply new coping strategies. Termination of regular therapy sessions provides clients the opportunity to rely solely on themselves to maintain therapeutic gains. Therapists convey that clients have learned what they needed in therapy sessions and are ready to take the next step of continued practice on their own. Rather than abruptly ending therapy sessions, therapists help clients plan carefully for upcoming therapy termination. Therapists review client progress and the key concepts underlying treatment success. The critical role of continued practice is emphasized, and therapists and clients generate a specific written relapse prevention plan for clients to implement after therapy has ended. Sometimes therapy ends prematurely, before clients realize maximum therapy gains. Managed care settings, in which the number of sessions may be limited, or other practical constraints may force clients to end therapy before they otherwise would. Therapists can help clients prepare for termination in these cases as well and may provide clients a list of low-cost self-help options for continued progress. Readers are referred to Hazlett-Stevens (2007) for an in-depth discussion of therapy termination practices and associated empirical research support.

### *Review of Client Progress and Essential Information*

Therapists begin the termination process by inviting clients to reflect back on how far they have come over the course of treatment. Therapists might remind clients of initial symptom severity and functional impairment discussed during early assessment sessions. Clients also are asked about their views of the therapy process and reasons for change. What factors does the client consider most responsible for desired changes and therapy success? If the client attributes success only to the therapist or to concurrent medication, therapists probe for specific client behaviors and characteristics that made change possible. As clients articulate their current understanding of anxiety, worry, and avoidance behavior, therapists emphasize the main points covered in early psychoeducation sessions. Clients often enjoy reflecting back on the therapy process, discovering how cognitive and behavioral coping responses are becoming new habits.

## Continued Practice of Therapy Skills and Coping Responses

Therapists next ask clients how they might continue to implement therapy strategies once sessions end. Clients are reminded that newly developed skills and responses are similar to other types of skills: either they become easier and more automatic with practice or they deteriorate over time with neglect. Öst (1989) made this point with the analogy of driving a car. When a person first learns to drive and receives a driver's license, he or she must drive frequently in a variety of traffic situations to refine driving skills. If he or she only drives on occasion, driving skills do not develop much further. In this case, challenging driving situations will be especially difficult. Similarly, new therapy skills will strengthen further with repeated practice. New coping responses eventually become automatic and replace previous anxiety spiral habits. When particularly stressful life events occur, clients are ready to respond in useful and adaptive ways. Along these lines, clients are reminded that future anxiety-provoking events are to be expected. Future episodes of anxiety, even high anxiety, are part of life and cannot be avoided. These future instances can be interpreted as opportunities to practice new coping responses rather than as setbacks or evidence that therapy gains have been lost. Therapists also ask clients about any foreseeable situations that might present a heightened risk for relapse. Stressful times of year, such as during the winter holidays or in the spring as federal tax deadlines approach, are identified ahead of time as vulnerable periods. Clients can plan for times of stress by increasing formal relaxation practice and returning to the written forms for regular self-monitoring and thought tracking.

## Written Relapse Prevention Plans

As client appreciate the importance of continued practice and anticipate future high-risk situations, therapists encourage them to generate a concrete plan of action. Clients detail the specific steps they will implement once therapy sessions end. How does the client plan to continue frequent daily self-monitoring and coping skill application practice? Which relaxation strategies might clients want to practice on a weekly basis to maintain skills? Which newly adopted self-care or health behaviors, such as an exercise routine or attending a yoga class, does the client plan to continue? What future situations might be approached as additional exposure exercises? How might clients take advantage of unplanned opportunities to confront their fears?

Before the last therapy session, clients organize and write down these relapse prevention plan components. Ongoing daily activities, such as self-monitoring, worry postponement to a worry period, and applied relaxation practice, could be listed in one column. Weekly formal practice of progressive relaxation, diaphragmatic breathing, or coping imagery rehearsal of upcoming possible scenarios could be listed in a "continued practice" column. Any additional situational exposure assignments clients have not yet conducted could be added in the final column. Finally, clients should list all courses of action they will take if they notice a return of symptoms. Re-reading psychoeducation material, resuming use of structured self-monitoring and thought tracking forms, and increasing relaxation practice are all possible options. In addition, clients always could contact the therapist for additional "booster" sessions. Therapists should present future booster sessions as an effective way to offset the worsening of symptoms as soon as they first appear. Thus, clients should not feel they should wait until symptoms are severe before seeking therapist support. Alternatively, follow-up sessions can be scheduled ahead of time. Clients attend follow-up sessions regardless of how they are doing, simply to check in with their therapist. Follow-up sessions are spaced apart at increasing time intervals, allowing therapist contacts to taper off gradually. Later follow-up contacts might involve brief telephone conversations in place of full-length office sessions.

## Early Termination of Therapy

When practical barriers to continued treatment sessions arise, therapists try to prepare clients for premature termination as much as possible. A practice plan for the therapy skills learned up to that point in treatment can help clients reap additional benefits once sessions have ended. Therapists also suggest how clients might continue to learn therapeutic strategies on their own. A list of specific cost-effective resources to clients, such as community center relaxation and stress management classes or local low-cost mental health clinics, should be provided. In addition, a few cognitive-behavioral self-help books targeting chronic worry and GAD have appeared on the market recently. The self-help material most consistent with the treatment described in this book can be found in *Women who worry too much* (Hazlett-Stevens 2005). Although targeted toward a female audience, the self-help exercises presented in each chapter apply to men and women equally. A similar cognitive-behavioral approach is described in a self-help book written for both sexes: *The worry cure* (Leahy 2005a). Finally, CBT procedures developed by Barlow and colleagues were recently updated and appear in their second edition *Mastery of your anxiety and worry* (MAW-2) Client Workbook (Craske & Barlow 2006a). Although the MAW-2 materials originally were designed to supplement therapist-guided treatment, the Client Workbook contains accessible psychoeducation information, worksheets, forms, and step-by-step client exercises.

## Chapter Summary

A variety of complications may arise over the course of treatment. Often these problems emerge in the form of non-compliance with self-monitoring or other home assignments. Clients may express reluctance to try assigned therapy activities between sessions. Clients also may return to session reporting they were unable to attempt or to complete assignments as planned. When homework compliance difficulties arise, therapists consider possible reasons including low client motivation, practical barriers, fear of increased anxiety, and a ruptured therapeutic alliance. Therapists respond to signs of low motivation by empathizing with client ambivalence, ensuring clients understand and accept the treatment rationale, and suggesting that clients view the time and effort required as an investment. Motivational enhancement techniques target these problems directly, and the two-chair experiential therapy technique might be used to explore sources of client ambivalence. Practical barriers are addressed with collaborative problem-solving. Clients having difficulty remembering to self-monitor might utilize external reminder cues such as post-it notes. Clients struggling to manage their time effectively may benefit from supplemental time management exercises that improve efficiency. When clients resist home assignments out of fear that their symptoms will worsen, therapists invite clients to view their prediction as an experiment to be tested and to examine beliefs that clients cannot tolerate discomfort. Unfavorable client perceptions of the therapy relationship and negative feelings toward therapists also impede the therapy process. In these cases, therapists empathize with clients, acknowledge their own contribution to the interaction, and encourage clients to speak freely about their feelings toward the therapist.

Complications specific to the different therapy techniques occur as well. During relaxation training procedures, clients may experience a paradoxical increase in anxiety. Clients may exhibit trouble at any stage of the cognitive therapy process. For example, clients may report initial difficulty determining whether a concrete problem can be solved or whether worry should be postponed to a worry period. Supplemental problem-solving interventions may be warranted. Clients unable to bring the mind back to the present moment after postponing a worry might benefit from supplemental mindfulness practice. Clients also may report difficulty with the cognitive techniques of generating alternative interpretations and predictions, examining the evidence, and decatastrophizing. Client demands for certainty may be addressed with supplemental therapy strategies that aim to increase tolerance of uncertainty (Dugas & Robichaud 2007). In addition, supplemental emotional deepening techniques may help restructure underlying core beliefs. Finally, therapists should watch for any client coping self-statements that are overly positive rather than balanced and flexible.

Superficial and one-dimensional statements of reassurance easily can become a new form of covert safety behavior that will undermine previous cognitive therapy efforts. In this case, therapists help clients generate more balanced and useful coping self-statements. Therapists also direct clients to take each anxious thought through the full thought tracking process before applying the new perspective. Problematic client responses during response prevention and *in vivo* exposure exercises should be expected and can inform future behavior therapy assignments.

Therapists help their clients prepare for upcoming therapy termination with relapse prevention strategies. Therapists encourage clients to reflect back on the therapy process and to assess their progress. Essential psychoeducation information is reviewed, and the importance of continued practice to maintain therapy gains is emphasized. Therapists and clients then generate a written relapse prevention plan for clients to follow after therapy sessions end. These plans typically contain methods for continued daily self-monitoring, worry postponement, and applied relaxation. A schedule for formal relaxation skill practice, additional response prevention or *in vivo* exposure exercises, and imagery exposure scenes is also set. Clients consider how they might respond to anticipated and unexpected stressful situations or a return of symptoms. Options such as increased formal practice, use of written therapy forms, and booster therapy sessions are listed. Therapists also might schedule infrequent follow-up therapy sessions or phone contacts to ensure continued client progress. When early termination occurs, clients might benefit from a similar plan consisting of continued practice and pursuit of additional treatment strategies on their own.

# References

Abel, J.L., & Borkovec, T.D. (1995). Generalizability of DSM-III-R generalized anxiety disorders to proposed DSM-IV criteria and cross-validation of proposed changes. *Journal of Anxiety Disorders, 9,* 303–315.

Abramson, L.Y., Seligman, M.E.P., & Teasdale, J.D. (1978). Learned helplessness in humans: Critique and reformulation. *Journal of Abnormal Psychology, 87,* 49–74.

Alden, L.E., Wiggins, J.S., & Pincus, A.L. (1990). Construction of circumplex scales for the Inventory of Interpersonal Problems. *Journal of Personality Assessment, 55,* 521–536.

Alwahhabi, F. (2003). Anxiety symptoms and generalized anxiety disorder in the elderly: A review. *Harvard Review of Psychiatry, 11,* 180–193.

American Psychiatric Association. (1952). *Diagnostic and statistical manual of mental disorders.* Washington, DC: Author.

American Psychiatric Association. (1968). *Diagnostic and statistical manual of mental disorders* (2nd ed.). Washington, DC: Author.

American Psychiatric Association. (1980). *Diagnostic and statistical manual of mental disorders* (3rd ed.). Washington, DC: Author.

American Psychiatric Association. (1987). *Diagnostic and statistical manual of mental disorders* (3rd ed. Revised). Washington, DC: Author.

American Psychiatric Association. (1994). *Diagnostic and statistical manual of mental disorders* (4th ed.). Washington, DC: Author.

American Psychiatric Association. (2000). *Diagnostic and statistical manual of mental disorders* (4th ed. Text Revision.). Washington, DC: Author.

Amir, N., Cashman, L., & Foa, E.B. (1997). Strategies of thought control in obsessive compulsive disorder. *Behaviour Research and Therapy, 35,* 775–777.

Andrews, G., & Peters, L. (1998). The psychometric properties of the Composite International Diagnostic Interview. *Social Psychiatry and Psychiatric Epidemiology, 33,* 80–88.

Antony, M.M., Orsillo, S.M., & Roemer, L.D. (2001). *Practitioner's guide to empirically based measures of anxiety.* Netherlands: Kluwer Academic.

Arntz, A. (2003). Cognitive therapy versus applied relaxation as treatment of generalized anxiety disorder. *Behaviour Research and Therapy, 41,* 633–646.

Barlow, D.H. (1988). *Anxiety and its disorders.* New York: Guilford Press.

Barlow, D.H., & Craske, M.G. (2006). *Mastery of your anxiety and panic: Client workbook* (4th ed.). New York: Oxford University Press.

Barlow, D.H., Rapee, R.M., & Brown, T.A. (1992). Behavioral treatment of generalized anxiety disorder. *Behavior Therapy, 23,* 551–570.

Barrowclough, C., King, P., Colville, J., Russell, E., Burns, A., & Tarrier, N. (2001). A randomized trial of the effectiveness of cognitive-behavioral therapy and supportive counseling for anxiety symptoms in older adults. *Journal of Consulting and Clinical Psychology, 69,* 756–762.

Basco, M.R. (2000). *Never good enough: How to use perfectionism to your advantage without ruining your life.* Carmichael, CA: Touchstone Books.

Beck, J.G., & Averill, P.M. (2004). Older adults. In R.G. Heimberg, C.L. Turk, & D.S. Mennin (Eds.), *Generalized anxiety disorder: Advances in research and practice* (pp. 409–433). New York: Guilford Press.

Beck, A.T., Emery, G., & Greenberg, R.L. (1985). *Anxiety disorders and phobias: A cognitive perspective.* New York: Basic Books.

Beck, A.T., Rush, A., Shaw, B., & Emery, G. (1979). *Cognitive therapy of depression.* New York: Guilford Press.

Beck, J.G., Stanley, M.A., & Zebb, B.J. (1995). Psychometric properties of the Penn State Worry Questionnaire in older adults. *Journal of Clinical Geropsychology, 1,* 33–42.

Beck, J.G., Stanley, M.A., & Zebb, B.J. (1996). Characteristics of generalized anxiety disorder in older adults: A descriptive study. *Behaviour Research and Therapy, 34,* 225–234.

Beck, J.G., Stanley, M.A., & Zebb, B.J. (1999). Effectiveness of the Hamilton Anxiety Rating Scale with older generalized anxiety disorder patients. *Journal of Clinical Geropsychology, 5,* 281–290.

Beck, A.T., & Steer, R.A. (1987). *Manual for the Beck Depression Inventory.* San Antonio, TX: The Psychological Corporation.

Beck, A.T., & Steer, R.A. (1990). *Beck Anxiety Inventory manual.* San Antonio, TX: The Psychological Corporation.

Beekman, A.T.F., Bremmer, M.A., Deeg, D.J.H., van Balkom, A.J.L.M., Snut, J.H., de Beurs, E., van Dyck, R., & van Tilburg, W. (1998). Anxiety disorders in later life: A report from the longitudinal aging study Amsterdam. *International Journal of Geriatric Psychiatry, 13,* 717–726.

Behar, E., Alcaine, O., Zuellig, A.R., & Borkokec, T.D. (2003). Screening for generalized anxiety disorder using the Penn State Worry Questionnaire: A receiver operating characteristic analysis. *Journal of Behavior Therapy and Experimental Psychiatry, 34,* 25–43.

Bernstein, D.A., & Borkovec, T.D. (1973). *Progressive relaxation training: A manual for the helping professions.* Champaign, IL: Research Press.

Bernstein, D.A., Borkovec, T.D., & Hazlett-Stevens, H. (2000). *New directions in progressive relaxation training: A guidebook for helping professionals.* Westport, CT: Greenwood Publishing.

Bhagwanjee, A., Parekh, A., Paruk, Z., Petersen, I., & Subedar, H. (1998). Prevalence of minor psychiatric disorders in an adult African rural community in South Africa. *Psychological Medicine, 28,* 1137–1147.

Bijl, R.V., Ravelli, A., Van Zessen, G. (1998). Prevalence of psychiatric disorder in the general population: Results of the Netherlands Mental Health Survey and Incidence Study (NEMESIS). *Social Psychiatry and Psychiatric Epidemiology, 33,* 587–595.

Blazer, D.G. (1997). Generalized anxiety disorder and panic disorder in the elderly: A review. *Harvard Review of Psychiatry, 5,* 18–27.

Blazer, D.G., Hughes, D., George, L.K., Schwartz, M., & Boyer, R. (1991). Generalized anxiety disorder. In L.N. Robins & D.A. Regier (Eds.), *Psychiatric disorders in America* (pp. 180–203) New York: Free Press.

Borkovec, T.D. (1979). Extensions of two-factor theory: Cognitive avoidance and autonomic perception. In N. Birbaumer & H.D. Kimmel (Eds.), *Biofeedback and self-regulation* (pp. 139–148). Hillsdale, NJ: Erlbaum.

Borkovec, T.D. (1994). The nature, functions, and origins of worry. In G.C.L. Davey & F. Tallis (Eds.), *Worrying: Perspectives on theory, assessment, and treatment* (pp. 5–34). New York: Wiley.

Borkovec, T.D. (2002). Life in the future versus life in the present. *Clinical Psychology: Science and Practice, 9,* 76–80.

Borkovec, T.D., Alcaine, O.M., & Behar, E. (2004). Avoidance theory of worry in generalized anxiety disorder. In R.G. Heimberg, C.L. Turk, & D.S. Mennin (Eds.), *Generalized anxiety disorder: Advances in research and practice* (pp. 3–28). New York: Guilford Press.

Borkovec, T.D., & Costello, E. (1993). Efficacy of applied relaxation and cognitive-behavioral therapy in the treatment of generalized anxiety disorder. *Journal of Consulting and Clinical Psychology, 61,* 611–619.

Borkovec, T.D., Hazlett-Stevens, H., & Diaz, M.L. (1999). The role of positive beliefs about worry in generalized anxiety disorder and its treatment. *Clinical Psychology and Psychotherapy, 6,* 126–138.

Borkovec, T.D., & Hu, S. (1990). The effect of worry on cardiovascular response to phobic imagery. *Behaviour Research and Therapy, 28,* 69–73.

Borkovec, T.D., & Inz, J. (1990). The nature of worry in generalized anxiety disorder: A predominance of thought activity. *Behaviour Research and Therapy, 28,* 153–158.

Borkovec, T.D., Lyonfields, J.D., Wiser, S.L., & Diehl, L. (1993). The role of worrisome thinking in the suppression of cardiovascular response to phobic imagery. *Behaviour Research and Therapy, 31,* 321–324.

Borkovec, T.D., & Mathews, A.M. (1988). Treatment of nonphobic anxiety disorders: A comparison of nondirective, cognitive, and coping desensitization therapy. *Journal of Consulting and Clinical Psychology, 56,* 877–884.

Borkovec, T.D., Mathews, A.M., Chambers, A., Ebrahimi, S., Lytle, R., & Nelson, R. (1987). The effects of relaxation training with cognitive or nondirective therapy and the role of relaxation-induced anxiety in the treatment of generalized anxiety. *Journal of Consulting and Clinical Psychology, 55,* 883–888.

Borkovec, T.D., Newman, M.G., & Castonguay, L.G. (2003). Cognitive-behavioral therapy for generalized anxiety disorder with integrations from interpersonal and experiential therapies. *CNS Spectrums, 8,* 382–389.

Borkovec, T.D., Newman, M.G., Pincus, A.L., & Lytle, R. (2002). A component analysis of cognitive-behavioral therapy for generalized anxiety disorder and the role of interpersonal problems. *Journal of Consulting and Clinical Psychology, 70,* 288–298.

Borkovec, T.D., & Roemer, L. (1995). Perceived functions of worrying among generalized anxiety disorder subjects: Distraction from more emotionally distressing topics? *Journal of Behavioral Therapy and Experimental Psychiatry, 26,* 25–30.

Borkovec, T.D., & Ruscio, A.M. (2001). Psychotherapy for generalized anxiety disorder. *Journal of clinical Psychiatry, 62,* 37–42.

Borkovec, T.D., & Whisman, M.A. (1996). Psychosocial treatments for generalized anxiety disorder. In M. Mavissakalian, & R. Prien (Eds.), *Long-term treatment of anxiety disorders.* Washingon, DC: American Psychiatric Association.

Borkovec, T.D., Wilkinson, L., Folensbee, R., & Lerman, C. (1983). Stimulus control applications to the treatment of worry. *Behaviour Research and Therapy, 21,* 247–251.

Brawman-Mintzer, O., Lydiard, R.B., Emmanuel, N., Payeur, R., Johnson, M., Roberts, J., Jarrell, M.P., & Ballenger, J.C. (1993). Psychiatric comorbidity in patients with generalized anxiety disorder. *American Journal of Psychiatry, 150,* 1216–1218.

Brown, T.A. (2003). Confirmatory factor analysis of the Penn State Worry Questionnaire: Multiple factors or method effects? *Behaviour Research and Therapy, 41,* 1411–1426.

Brown, T.A., Antony, M.M., & Barlow, D.H. (1992). Psychometric properties of the Penn State Worry Questionnaire in a clinical anxiety disorders sample. *Behaviour Research and Therapy, 30,* 33–37.

Brown, T.A., & Barlow, D.H. (1992). Comorbidity among anxiety disorders: Implications for treatment and DSM-IV. *Journal of Consulting and Clinical Psychology, 60,* 835–844.

Brown, T.A., & Barlow, D.H. (2002). Classification of anxiety and mood disorders. In D.H. Barlow (Ed.) *Anxiety and its disorders: The nature and treatment of anxiety and panic* (pp. 292–327). New York: Guilford Press.

Brown, T.A., Barlow, D.H., & Liebowitz, M.R. (1994). The empirical basis of generalized anxiety disorder. *American Journal of Psychiatry, 151,* 1272–1280.

Brown, T.A., DiNardo, P.A., & Barlow, D.H. (1994). *Anxiety Disorders Interview Schedule for DSM-IV (ADIS-IV).* Albany, NY: Graywind.

Brown, T.A., DiNardo, P.A., Lehman, C.L., & Campbell, L.A. (2001). Reliability of DSM-IV anxiety and mood disorders: Implications for the classification of emotional disorders. *Journal of Abnormal Psychology, 110,* 49–58.

Brown, T.A., O'Leary, T.A., & Barlow, D.H. (2001). Generalized anxiety disorder. In D.H. Barlow (Ed.), *Clinical handbook of psychological disorders: A step-by-step treatment manual* (3rd ed.). New York: Guilford Press.

Burns, D., & Auerbach, A. (1996). Therapeutic empathy in cognitive-behavioural therapy: Does it really make a difference? In P. Salkovskis (Ed.), *Frontiers of cognitive therapy* (pp. 135–164). New York: Guilford Press.

Butler, G., Fennell, M., Robson, P., & Gelder, M. (1991). Comparison of behavior therapy and cognitive behavior therapy in the treatment of generalized anxiety disorder. *Journal of Consulting and Clinical Psychology, 59,* 167–175.

Butler, G., Wells, A., & Dewick, H. (1995). Differential effects of worry and imagery after exposure to a stressful stimulus: A pilot study. *Behavioural and Cognitive Psychotherapy, 23,* 45–56.

Cartwright-Hatton, S., & Wells, A. (1997). Beliefs about worry and intrusions: The Meta Cognitions Questionnaire and its correlates. *Journal of Anxiety Disorders, 11,* 279–296.

Carver, C.S., & White, T.L. (1994). Behavioral inhibition, behavioral activation, and affective responses to impending reward and punishment: The BIS/BAS Scales. *Journal of Personality and Social Psychology, 67,* 319–333.

Cassidy, J. (1995). Attachment and generalized anxiety disorder. In D. Cicchetti & S. Toth (Eds.), *Rochester Symposium on Developmental Psychopathology: Vol. 6. Emotion, cognition and representation* (pp. 343–370). Rochester, NY: University of Rochester Press.

Cohen, J. (1988). *Statistical power analysis for the behavioral sciences.* San Diego, CA: Academic Press.

Costa, P.T., Jr., & McCrae, R.R. (1992). *NEO PI-R: Professional manual.* Odessa, FL: Psychological Assessment Resources, Inc.

Craske, M.G., & Barlow, D.H. (2006a). *Mastery of your anxiety and worry: Client workbook* (2nd ed.). New York: Oxford University Press.

Craske, M.G., & Barlow, D.H. (2006b). *Mastery of your anxiety and panic: Therapist guide* (4th ed.). New York: Oxford University Press.

Craske, M.G., Barlow, D.H., & O'Leary, T. (1992). *Mastery of Your Anxiety and Worry.* San Antonio, TX: Psychological Corporation.

Craske, M.G., & Hazlett-Stevens, H. (2002). Facilitating symptom reduction and behavior change in GAD: The issue of control. *Clinical Psychology: Research and Practice, 9,* 69–75.

Craske, M.G., Rapee, R.M., Jackel, L., & Barlow, D.H. (1989). Qualitative dimensions of worry in DSM-III-R generalized anxiety disorder subjects and nonanxious controls. *Behaviour Research and Therapy, 27,* 397–402.

Crits-Christoph, P., Connolly, M.B., Azarian, K., Crits-Christoph, K., & Shappell, S. (1996). An open trial of brief supportive-expressive psychotherapy in the treatment of generalized anxiety disorder. *Psychotherapy: Theory, Research, Practice, Training, 33,* 418–430.

Crits-Christoph, P., Crits-Christoph, K., Wolf-Palacio, D., Fichter, M., & Rudick, D. (1995). Brief supportive-expressive psychodynamic therapy for generalized anxiety disorder. In J.P. Barber & P. Crits-Christoph (Eds.), *Dynamic therapies for psychiatric disorders (Axis I)* (pp. 43–83). New York: Basic Books.

Davey, G.C.L. (1994). Pathological worrying as exacerbated problem solving. In G.C.L. Davey, & F. Tallis (Eds.), *Worrying: Perspectives on theory, assessment and treatment* (pp. 35–61). New York: Wiley.

Davey, G.C.L., & Levy, S. (1998). Catastrophic worrying: Personal inadequacy and a perseverative iterative style as features of the catastrophizing process. *Journal of Abnormal Psychology, 107,* 576–586.

Davey, G.C.L., Tallis, F., & Capuzzo, N. (1996). Beliefs about the consequences of worrying. *Cognitive Therapy and Research, 20,* 499–520.

Davis, R.N., & Valentiner, D.P. (2000). Does meta-cognitive theory enhance our understanding of pathological worry and anxiety? *Personality and Individual Differences, 29,* 513–526.

D'Errico, G.M., Galassi, J.P., Schanberg, R., & Ware, W.B. (1999). Development and validation of the Cancer Worries Inventory: A measure of illness-related cognitions. *Journal of Psychosocial Oncology, 17,* 119–137.

Di Nardo, P.A., Moras, K., Barlow, D.H., Rapee, R.M., & Brown, T.A. (1993). Reliability of DSM-III-R anxiety disorder categories: Using the Anxiety Disorders Interview Schedule-Revised (ADIS-R). *Archives of General Psychiatry, 50,* 251–256.

DiNardo, P.A., Brown, T.A., & Barlow, D.H. (1994). *Anxiety Disorders Interview Schedule for DSM-IV: Lifetime Version (ADIS-IV-L).* Albany, NY: Graywind.

Drews, A.A., & Hazlett-Stevens, H. 2008. Relationships between irritable bowel syndrome, generalized anxiety disorder, and worry-related constructs. *International Journal of Clinical and Health Psychology.* Volume 8.

Dugas, M.J., Buhr, K., & Ladouceur, R. (2004). The role of intolerance of uncertainty in etiology and maintenance. In R.G. Heimberg, C.L. Turk, & D.S. Mennin (Eds.), *Generalized anxiety disorder: Advances in research and practice* (pp. 3–28). New York: Guilford Press.

Dugas, M.J., Gagnon, F., Ladouceur, R., & Freeston, M.H. (1998). Generalized anxiety disorder: A preliminary test of a conceptual model. *Behaviour Research and Therapy, 36,* 216–226.

Dugas, M.J., Gosselin, P., & Ladouceur, R. (2001). Intolerance of uncertainty and worry: Investigating specificity in a nonclinical sample. *Cognitive Therapy and Research, 25,* 551–558.

Dugas, M.J., Ladouceur, R., Léger, E., Freeston, M.H., Langlois, F., Provencher, M.D., & Boisvert, J.M. (2003). Group cognitive-behavioral therapy for generalized anxiety disorder: Treatment outcome and long-term follow-up. *Journal of Consulting and Clinical Psychology, 71,* 821–825.

Dugas, M.J., & Robichaud, M. (2007). *Cognitive-behavioral treatment for generalized anxiety disorder: From science to practice.* New York: Routledge/Taylor & Francis.

Ellis, A. (1962). *Reason and Emotion in Psychotherapy.* New York: Lyle Stuart.

Eysenck, H.J., & Eysenck, S.B.G. (1975). *Eysenck Personality Questionnaire.* San Diego, CA: Educational and Industrial Testing Service.

Faravelli, C., Degl'Innocenti, B.G., & Giardinelli, L. (1989). Epidemiology of anxiety disorders in Florence. *Acta Psychiatrica Scandinavica, 79,* 308–312.

First, M.B., Spitzer, R.L., Gibbon, M., & Williams, J.B.W. (2001). *Structured clinical interview for DSM-IV axis I disorders.* New York: Biometrics Research Department, New York State Psychiatric Institute.

Francis, K., & Dugas, M.J. (2004). Assessing positive beliefs about worry: Validation of a structured interview. *Personality and Individual Differences, 37,* 405–415.

Freeston, M.H., Dugas, M.J., & Ladouceur, R. (1996). Thoughts, images, worry and anxiety. *Cognitive Therapy and Research, 20,* 265–273.

Freeston, M.H., Rhéaume, J., Letarte, H., Dugas, M.J., & Ladouceur, R. (1994). Why do people worry? *Personality and Individual Differences, 17,* 791–802.

Fresco, D.M., Heimberg, R.G., Mennin, D.S., & Turk, C.L. (2002). Confirmatory factor analysis of the Penn State Worry Questionnaire. *Behaviour Research and Therapy, 40,* 313–323.

Fresco, D.M., Mennin, D.S., Heimberg, R.G., & Turk, C.L. (2003). Using the Penn State Worry Questionnaire to identify individuals with generalized anxiety disorder: A receiver operating characteristic analysis. *Journal of Behavior Therapy and Experimental Psychiatry, 34,* 283–291.

Frisch, M.B. (1994). *Quality of Life Inventory: Manual and treatment guide.* Minneapolis, MN: National Computer Systems.

Fruzzetti, A.E., Shenk, C., Mosco, E., & Lowry, K. (2003). Emotion regulation. In W.T. O'Donohue, J.E. Fisher, & S.C. Hayes (Eds.), *Cognitive behavior therapy: Applying empirically supported techniques in your practice* (pp. 152–159). New York: John Wiley & Sons.

Fyer, A.J., Endicott, J., Mannuzza, S., & Klein, D.F. (1995). *Schedule for Affective Disorders and Schizophrenia-Lifetime Version, modified for the study of anxiety disorders, updated for DSM-IV (SADS-LA-IV).* Unpublished measure, Anxiety Genetics Unit, New York State Psychiatric Institute, New York, NY.

Garry, M., Manning, C.G., & Loftus, E.F. (1996). Imagination inflation: Imagining a childhood event inflates confidence that it occurred. *Psychonomic Bulletin & Review, 3,* 208–214.

Gillis, M.M., Haaga, D.A.F., Ford, G.T. (1995). Normative values for the Beck Anxiety Inventory, Fear Questionnaire, Penn State Worry Questionnaire, and Social Phobia and Anxiety Inventory. *Psychological Assessment, 7,* 450–455.

Goldfried, M.R. (1971). Systematic desensitization as training in self-control. *Journal of Consulting and Clinical Psychology, 37,* 228–234.

Goldfried, M.R. (1996). *Cognitive-affective behavior therapy* (video-tape). Washington, DC: American Psychological Association.

Gorenstein, E.E., Kleber, M.S., Mohlman, J., DeJesus, M., Gorman, J.M., & Papp, L.A. (2005). Cognitive-behavioral therapy for management of anxiety and medication taper in older adults. *American Journal of Geriatric Psychiatry, 13,* 901–909.

Gosselin, P., Langlois, F., Freeston, M.H., Ladouceur, R., Dugas, M.J., & Pelletier, O. (2002). Le Questionnaire d'évitement cognitif (QEC): Développement et validation auprès d'adultes et d'adolescents [The Cognitive Avoidance Questionnaire (CAQ): Development and validation among adult and adolescent samples] *Journal de Thérapie Comportementale et Cognitive, 12,* 24–37.

Gould, R.A., Otto, M.W., Pollack, M.P., & Yap, L. (1997). Cognitive-behavioral and pharmacological treatment of generalized anxiety disorder: A preliminary meta analysis. *Behavior Therapy, 28,* 285–305.

Gould, R.A., Safren, S.A., Washington, D., & Otto, M.W. (2004). A meta-analytic review of cognitive-behavioral treatments. In R.G. Heimberg, C.L. Turk, & D.S. Mennin (Eds.), *Generalized anxiety disorder: Advances in research and practice* (pp. 284–264). New York: Guilford Press.

Graham, J.R. (2006). MMPI-*2: Assessing personality and psychopathology* (4th ed.). New York: Oxford University Press.

Gratz, K.L., & Roemer, L. (2004). Multidimensional assessment of emotion regulation and dysregulation: Development, factor structure, and initial validation of the Difficulties in Emotion Regulation Scale. *Journal of Psychopathology and Behavioral Assessment, 26,* 41–54.

Green, J.M., Kafetsios, K., Statham, H.E., & Snowdon, C.M. (2003). Factor Structure, Validity and Reliability of the Cambridge Worry Scale in a Pregnant Population. *Journal of Health Psychology, 8,* 753–764.

Greenberg, L., Rice, L., & Elliott, R. (1996). *Facilitating emotional change: The moment by moment process.* New York: Guilford Press.

Greenberg, L.S., & Safran, J.D. (1987). *Emotion in Psychotherapy.* New York: Guilford Press.

Hamilton, M. (1959). The assessment of anxiety states by rating. *British Journal of Psychiatry, 32,* 50–55.

Hamilton, M. (1960). A rating scale for depression. *Journal of Neurology, Neurosurgery and Psychiatry, 23,* 56–62.

Hayes, S.C., Strosahl, K., & Wilson, K.G. (1999). *Acceptance and Commitment Therapy: An Experimental Approach to Behavior Change.* New York: Guilford Press.

Hazlett, R.L., McLeod, D.R., & Hoehn-Saric, R. (1994). Muscle tension in generalized anxiety disorder: Elevated muscle tonus or agitated movement? *Psychophysiology, 31,* 189–195.

Hazlett-Stevens, H. (1997, November). *Cognitive flexibility in an analog generalized anxiety disorder population.* Poster presented at the 31st Annual Convention of the Association for Advancement of Behavior Therapy, Miami, FL.

Hazlett-Stevens, H. (2000, September). *Cognitive flexibility deficits in generalized anxiety disorder.* Poster presented at the 30th annual meeting of the European Association for Behavioral and Cognitive Therapies (EABCT), Granada, Spain.

Hazlett-Stevens, H. (2005). *Women who worry too much: How to stop worry and anxiety from ruining relationships, work, and fun.* Oakland, CA: New Harbinger Publications.

Hazlett-Stevens, H. (2007). Termination with patients with anxiety disorders. To appear in W.T. O'Donohue & M.A. Cucciare (Eds.), *A clinician's guide to the theory and practice of termination in psychotherapy.* New York: Routledge/Taylor & Francis.

Hazlett-Stevens, H., & Craske, M.G. (2003a). Breathing retraining and diaphragmatic breathing techniques. In W. O'Donohue, J.E. Fisher, & S.C. Hayes (Eds.), *Cognitive behavior therapy: Applying empirically supported techniques in your practice.* New York: Wiley.

Hazlett-Stevens, H., & Craske, M.G. (2003b). The catastrophizing worry process in generalized anxiety disorder: A preliminary investigation of an analog population. *Behavioural and Cognitive Psychotherapy, 31,* 387–401.

Hazlett-Stevens, H., Craske, M.G., Mayer, E.A., Chang, L., & Naliboff, B.D. (2003). Prevalence of irritable bowel syndrome among university students: The roles of worry, neuroticism, anxiety sensitivity, and visceral anxiety. *Journal of Psychosomatic Research, 55,* 501–505.

Hazlett-Stevens, H., Ullman, J.B., Craske, M.G. (2004). Factor Structure of the Penn State Worry Questionnaire: Examination of a Method Factor. *Assessment, 11,* 361–370.

Hazlett-Stevens, H., Zucker, B.G., Craske, M.G. (2002). The relationship of thought-action fusion to pathological worry and generalized anxiety disorder. *Behaviour Research and Therapy, 40,* 1199–1204.

Heimberg, R.G., Turk, C.L., & Mennin, D.S. (2004). *Generalized anxiety disorder: Advances in research and practice.* New York: Guilford Press.

Hertzsprung, E.A., Konnert, C., & Brinker, J. (2004). Research note: Development of a Worry Questionnaire for Nursing Home Residents. *Canadian Journal on Aging, 23,* 359–366.

Hoehn-Saric, R., Hazlett, R.L., & McLeod, D.R. (1993). Generalized anxiety disorder with early and late onset of anxiety symptoms. *Comprehensive Psychiatry, 34,* 291–298.

Hoehn-Saric, R., McLeod, D.R., & Zimmerli, W.D. (1989). Symptoms and treatment responses of generalized anxiety disorder patients with high versus low levels of cardiovascular complaints. *American Journal of Psychiatry, 146,* 854–859.

Horney, K. (1950). *Neurosis and human growth: The struggle toward self-realization.* New York: W.W. Norton.

Hunt, S., Wisocki, P., & Yanko, J. (2003). Worry and use of coping strategies among older and younger adults. *Journal of Anxiety Disorders, 17,* 547–560.

Jacobson, E. (1934). *You must relax.* New York: McGraw-Hill.

Jacobson, E. (1938). *Progressive relaxation.* Chicago: University of Chicago press.

Joorman, J., & Stöber, J. (1997). Measuring facets of worry: A LISREL analysis of the Worry Domains Questionnaire. *Personality and Individuals Differences, 23,* 827–837.

Junginger, J., Phelan, E., Cherry, K., & Levy, J. (1993). Prevalence of psychopathology in elderly persons in nursing homes and in the community. *Hospital & Community Psychiatry, 44,* 381–383.

Kabat-Zinn, J. (1990). *Full Catastrophe Living: Using the Wisdom of your Mind to Face Stress, Pain and Illness.* New York: Dell Publishing.

Kabat-Zinn, J. (1994). *Wherever you go there you are.* New York: Hyperion.

Kabat-Zinn, J., Massion, A.O., Kristeller, J., Peterson, L.G., Fletcher, K., Pbert, L., Linderking, W., & Santorelli, S.F. (1992). Effectiveness of a meditation-based stress reduction program in the treatment of anxiety disorders. *American Journal of Psychiatry, 149,* 936–943.

Kessler, R.C., Berglund, P., Demler, O., Jin, R., Merikangas, K.R., & Walters, E.E. (2005). Lifetime prevalence of age-of-onset distributions of DSM-IV disorders in the National Comorbidity Survey Replication. *Archives of General Psychiatry, 62,* 593–602.

Kessler, R.C., Chiu, W.T., Demler, O., & Walters, E.E. (2005). Prevalence, severity, and comorbidity of 12-month DSM-IV disorders in the National Comorbidity Survey Replication. *Archives of General Psychiatry, 62,* 617–627.

Kessler, R.C., McGonagle, K.A., Zhao, S., Nelson, C.B., Hughes, M., Eshleman, S., Wittchen, H.U., & Kendler, K.S. (1994). Lifetime and 12-month prevalence of DSM-III-R psychiatric disorders in the United States: Results from the National Comorbidity Study. *Archives of General Psychiatry, 51,* 8–19.

Klosko, J.S., & Sanderson, W.C. (1999). *Cognitive-behavioral treatment of depression.* Northvale, NJ: Jason Aronson Inc.

Kobak, K.A., Taylor, L.H., Dottl, S.L., Greist, J.H., Jefferson, J.W., Burroughs, D., Mantle, J.M., Katzelnick, D.J., Norton, R., Henk, H.J., & Serlin, R.C. (1997). A computer-administered telephone interview to identify mental disorders. *Journal of the American Medial Association, 278,* 905–910.

Kohlenberg, R.J. & Tsai, M. (1991). *Functional Analytic Psychotherapy: Creating intense and curative therapeutic relationships*. New York: Plenum.

Ladouceur, R., Blais, F., Freeston, M.H., & Dugas, M.J. (1998). Problem solving and problem orientation in generalized anxiety disorder. *Journal of Anxiety Disorders, 12,* 139–152.

Ladouceur, R., Dugas, M.J., Freeston, M.H., Léger, E., Gagnon, F., & Thibodeau, N. (2000). Efficacy of a cognitive-behavioral treatment for generalized anxiety disorder: Evaluation in a controlled clinical trial. *Journal of Consulting and Clinical Psychology, 68,* 957–964.

Ladoucer, R., Dugas, M.J., Freeston, M.H., Rhéaume, J., Blais, F., Boisert, J.M., Gagnon, F., & Thibodeau, N. (1999). Specificity of generalized anxiety disorder symptoms and processes. *Behavior Therapy, 30,* 191–207.

Ladouceur, R., Léger, E., Dugas, M., & Freeston, M.H. (2004). Cognitive-behavioral treatment of Generalized Anxiety Disorder (GAD) for older adults. *International Psychogeriatrics, 16,* 195–207.

Le Roux, H., Gatz, M., & Wetherell, J.L. (2005). Age at onset of generalized anxiety disorder in older adults. *American Journal of Geriatric Psychology, 13,* 23–30.

Leahy, R.L. (2004). Cognitive-behavioral therapy. In R.G. Heimberg, C.L. Turk, & D.S. Mennin (Eds.), *Generalized anxiety disorder: Advances in research and practice* (pp. 265–292). New York: Guilford Press.

Leahy, R.L. (2005a). *The worry cure: Seven steps to stop worry from stopping you.* New York: Harmony Books.

Leahy, R.L. (2005b). Panic, agoraphobia, and generalized anxiety. In N. Kazantzis, F.P. Deane, K.R. Ronan, & L. L'Abate (Eds.), *Using homework assignments in cognitive behavior therapy* (pp. 193–218). New York: Routledge/Taylor & Francis.

Leahy, R.L., & Holland, S.J. (2000). *Treatment plans and interventions for depression and anxiety disorders.* New York: The Guilford Press.

Lehrer, P.M., Woolfolk, R.L. (1982). Self-report assessment of anxiety: Somatic, cognitive, and behavioral modalities. *Behavioral Assessment, 4,* 167–177.

Lewinsohn, P.M. (1975). Engagement in pleasant activities and depression levels. *Journal of Abnormal Psychology, 84,* 729–731.

Linehan, M.M. (1993). *Cognitive Behavioral Treatment of Borderline Personality Disorder.* New York: Guilford Press.

Lovibond, P.F., & Lovibond, S.H. (1995). The structure of negative emotional states: Comparison of the Depression Anxiety Stress Scales (DASS) with the Beck Depression and Anxiety Inventories. *Behaviour Research and Therapy, 33,* 335–343.

Luoma, J.B., & Hayes, S.C. (2003). Cognitive diffusion. In W.T. O'Donohue, J.E. Fisher, & S.C. Hayes (Eds.), *Cognitive behavior therapy: Applying empirically supported techniques in your practice* (pp 71–78). New York: John Wiley & Sons.

Lydiard, R.B. (1992). Anxiety and the irritable bowel syndrome. *Psychiatric Annals, 22,* 612–618.

Lyonfields, J.D., Borkovec, T.D., & Thayer, J.F. (1995). Vagal tone in generalized anxiety disorder and the effects of aversive imagery and worrisome thinking. *Behavior Therapy, 26,* 457–466.

MacLeod, C., & Rutherford, E. (2004). Information-processing approaches: Assessing the selective functioning of attention, interpretation, and retrieval. In R.G. Heimberg, C.L. Turk, & D.S. Mennin (Eds.), *Generalized anxiety disorder: Advances in research and practice* (pp. 109–142). New York: Guilford Press.

Martell, C.R. (2003). Behavioral activation therapy for depression. In W.T. O'Donohue, J.E. Fisher, & S.C. Hayes (Eds.), *Cognitive behavior therapy: Applying empirically supported techniques in your practice* (pp. 28–32). New York: John Wiley & Sons.

Marten, P.A., Brown, T.A., Barlow, D.H., Borkovec, T.D., Shear, M.K., Lydiard, R.B. (1993). Evaluation of the ratings comprising the associated symptom criterion of DSM-III-R generalized anxiety disorder. *Journal of Nervous and Mental Disease, 181,* 676–682.

McCabe, R.E., & Antony, M.M. (2005). Panic disorder and agoraphobia. In M.M. Antony, D.R. Ledley, & R.G. Heimberg (Eds.), *Improving outcomes and preventing relapse in cognitive-behavioral therapy* (pp. 1–37). New York: Guilford Press.

Medina-Mora, M.E., Borges, G., Lara, C., Benjet, C., Blanco, J., Feliz, C., Villatoro, J., Rojas, E., & Zambrano, J. (2005). Prevalence, service use, and demographic correlates of 12-month DSM-IV psychiatric disorders in Mexico: Results from the Mexican National Comorbidity Survey. *Psychological Medicine, 35,* 1–11.

Mendlowicz, M.V., & Stein, M.B. (2000). Quality of life in individuals with anxiety disorders. *American Journal of Psychiatry, 157,* 669–682.

Mennin, D.S. (2004). Emotion regulation therapy for generalized anxiety disorder. *Clinical Psychology and Psychotherapy, 11,* 17–29.

Mennin, D.S., Heimberg, R.G., & Turk, C.L. (2004). Clinical presentation and diagnostic features. In R.G. Heimberg, C.L. Turk, & D.S. Mennin (Eds.), *Generalized anxiety disorder: Advances in research and practice* (pp. 3–28). New York: Guilford Press.

Mennin, D.S., Heimberg, R.G., Turk, C.L., & Fresco, D.M. (2002). Applying an emotion regulation framework to integrative approaches to generalized anxiety disorder. *Clinical Psychology: Science and Practice, 9,* 85–90.

Mennin, D.S., Heimberg, R.G., Turk, C.L., & Fresco, D.M. (2005). Preliminary evidence for an emotion dysregulation model of generalized anxiety disorder. *Behaviour Research and Therapy, 43,* 1281–1310.

Mennin, D.S., Turk, C.L., Heimberg, R.G., & Carmin, C. (2004). Regulation of emotion in generalized anxiety disorder. In M.A. Reinecke and D.A. Clark (Eds.), *Cognitive therapy over the lifespan: Theory, research, and practice* (pp. 60–89). New York: Wiley.

Metzger, R.L., Miller, M., Cohen, M., Sofka, M., & Borkovec, T. (1990). Worry changes decision making: The effect of negative thoughts on cognitive processing. *Journal of Clinical Psychology, 46,* 78–88.

Meyer, T.J., Miller, M.L., Metzger, R.L., & Borkovec, T.D. (1990). Development and validation of the Penn State worry questionnaire. *Behaviour Research and Therapy, 28,* 487–494.

Miller, J.J., Fletcher, K., & Kabat-Zinn, J. (1995). Three-year follow-up and clinical implications of a mindfulness meditation-based stress reduction intervention in the treatment of anxiety disorders. *General Hospital Psychiatry, 17,* 192–200.

Miller, W.R., & Rollnick, S. (2002). *Motivational interviewing* (2nd ed.). New York: Guilford.

Mohlman, J., Gorenstein, E.E., Kleber, M., De Jesus, M., Gorman, J.M., & Papp, L.A. (2003). Standard and enhanced cognitive-behavior therapy for late-life generalized anxiety disorder: Two pilot investigations. *American Journal of Geriatric Psychiatry, 11,* 24–32.

Molina, S., & Borkovec, T.D. (1994). The Penn State Worry Questionnaire: Psychometric properties and associated characteristics. In G.C.L. Davey & F. Tallis (Eds.), *Worrying: Perspectives on theory, assessment, and treatment* (pp. 265–283). Chichester, UK: Wiley.

Mowrer, O.H. (1947). On the dual nature of learning a re-interpretation of "conditioning" and "problem-solving." *Harvard Educational Review, 17,* 102–148.

Newman, M.G. (2000). Generalized anxiety disorder. In M. Hersen & M. Biaggio (Eds.), *Effective brief therapies: A clinician's guide* (pp. 157–178). San Diego, CA: Academic Press.

Newman, M.G., Castonguay, L.G., Borkovec, T.D., & Molnar, C. (2004). Integrative therapy for generalized anxiety disorder. In R.G. Heimberg, C.L. Turk, & D.S. Mennin (Eds.), *Generalized anxiety disorder: Advances in research and practice* (pp. 320–350). New York: Guilford Press.

Newman, M.G., Zuellig, A.R., Kachin, K.E., Constantino, M.J., Przeworski, A., Erickson, T., & Cashman-McGrath, L. (2002). Preliminary reliability and validity of the Generalized Anxiety Disorder Questionnaire-IV: A revised self-report diagnostic measure of generalized anxiety disorder. *Behavior Therapy, 33,* 215–233.

Offord, D.R., Boyle, M.H., Campbell, D., Goring, P., Lin, E., Wrong, M., & Racine, A. (1996). One year prevalence of psychiatric disorder in Ontarians 15 to 64 years of age. *Canadian Journal of Psychiatry, 41,* 559–563.

Öst, L.G. (1987). Applied relaxation: Description of a coping technique and review of controlled studies. *Journal of Consulting and Clinical Psychology, 59,* 100–114.

Öst, L.G. (1989). A maintenance program for behavioral treatment of anxiety disorders. *Behaviour Research and Therapy, 27,* 123–130.

Öst, L.G., & Breitholtz, E. (2000). Applied relaxation vs. cognitive therapy in the treatment of generalized anxiety disorder. *Behaviour Research and Therapy, 38,* 777–790.

Parmelee, P.A., Katz, I.R., & Lawton, M.P. (1993). Anxiety and its association with depression among institutionalized elderly. *American Journal of Geriatric Psychiatry, 1,* 46–58.

Pincus, A.L., & Borkovec, T.D. (1994, June). *Interpersonal problems in generalized anxiety disorder: Preliminary clustering of patients' interpersonal dysfunction.* Paper presented at the annual meeting of the American Psychological Society, New York.

Pini, S., Cassano, G.B., Simonini, E., Savino, M., Russo, A., & Montomery, S.A. (1997). Prevalence of anxiety disorders comorbidity in bipolar depression, unipolar depression and dysthymia. *Journal of Affective Disorders, 42,* 145–153.

Rachman, S. (2004). *Anxiety* (2nd ed.). New York: Psychology Press Ltd.

Radley, M., Redston, C., Bates, F., Pontefract, M., Lindesay, J. (1997). Effectiveness of group anxiety management with elderly clients of a community psychogeriatric team. *International Journal of Geriatric Psychiatry, 12,* 79–84.

Rickard, H.C., Scogin, F., Keith, S. (1994). A one-year follow-up of relaxation training for elders with subjective anxiety. *Gerontologist, 34,* 121–122.

Ritter, M.R., & Hazlett-Stevens, H. (2006). The use of exposure and ritual prevention in the treatment of harm obsessions with covert compulsions. *Clinical Case Studies, 5,* 455–476.

Ritter, M.R., & Hazlett-Stevens, H. (in preparation). *An investigation of intolerance of uncertainty in worry using a gamble preference task.* Unpublished manuscript.

Robins, L.N., Cottler, L., Bucholz, K., & Compton, W. (1995). *The Diagnostic Interview Schedule, Version IV.* St. Louis, MO: Washington University Medical School.

Roemer, L. (2001a). Measures for anxiety and related constructs. In A.M. Anthony, S.M. Orsillo, & L. Roemer (Eds.), *Practitioner's guide to empirically based measures of anxiety* (pp. 49–83). Dordrecht, Netherlands: Kluwer Academic Publishers.

Roemer, L. (2001b). Measures for generalized anxiety disorder. In A.M. Anthony, S.M. Orsillo, & L. Roemer (Eds.), *Practitioner's guide to empirically based measures of anxiety* (pp. 49–83). Dordrecht, Netherlands: Kluwer Academic Publishers.

Roemer, L., Molina, S., & Borkovec, T.D. (1997). An investigation of worry content among generally anxious individuals. *The Journal of Nervous and Mental Disease, 185,* 314–319.

Roemer, L., Molina, S., Litz, B.T., & Borkovec, T.D. (1997). Preliminary investigation of the role of previous exposure to potentially traumatizing events in generalized anxiety disorder. *Depression and Anxiety, 4,* 134–138.

Roemer, L., Borkovec, M., Posa, S., & Borkovec, T.D. (1995). A self-report diagnostic measure of generalized anxiety disorder. *Journal of Behavior Therapy and Experimental Psychiatry, 26,* 345–350.

Roemer, L., & Orsillo, S.M. (2005). An acceptance based behavior therapy for generalized anxiety disorder. In S.M. Orsillo & L. Roemer (Eds.), *Acceptance and Mindfulness-based approaches to anxiety: Conceptualization and treatment.* New York: Springer.

Roemer, L., & Orsillo, S.M. (2007). An open trial of an acceptance-based behavior therapy for generalized anxiety disorder. *Behavior Therapy, 38,* 72–85.

Roemer, L., Orsillo, S.M., & Barlow, D.H. (2002). Generalized anxiety disorder. In D.H. Barlow (Ed), *Anxiety and its disorders: The nature and treatment of anxiety and panic* (pp. 477–515). New York: Guilford Press.

Roemer, L., Salters, K., Raffa, S., & Orsillo, S.M. (2005). Fear and avoidance of internal experiences in GAD: Preliminary tests of a conceptual model. *Cognitive Therapy and Research, 29,* 71–78.

Roy-Byrne, P.P., & Wagner, A. (2004). Primary care perspectives on generalized anxiety disorder. *Journal of Clinical Psychiatry, 65,* 20–26.

Ruscio, A.M. (2002). Delimiting the boundaries of generalized anxiety disorder: Differentiating high worriers with and without GAD. *Journal of Anxiety Disorders, 16,* 377–400.

Ruscio, A.M., Lane, M., Roy-Byrne, P., Stang, P.E., Stein, D.J., Wittchen, H., & Kessler, R.C. (2005). Should excessive worry be required for a diagnosis of generalized anxiety disorder? Results from the US National Comorbidity Survey Replication. *Psychological Medicine, 35,* 1–12.

Rygh, J.R., & Sanderson, W.C. (2004). *Treating generalized anxiety disorder: Evidence-based strategies, tools, and techniques.* New York: Guilford Press.

Safran, J., & Muran, J.C. (2000). *Negotiating the therapeutic alliance: A relational treatment guide.* New York: The Guilford Press.

Safran, J., & Segal, Z. (1990). *Interpersonal process in cognitive therapy.* New York: Basic Books.

Samilov, A., & Goldfried, M.R. (2000). Role of emotion in cognitive-behavior therapy. *Clinical Psychology: Science and Practice, 7,* 373–385.

Sanderson, W.C., & Barlow, D.H. (1990). A description of patients diagnosed with DSM-III-R generalized anxiety disorder. *Journal of Nervous and Mental Disease, 178,* 588–591.

Sanderson, W.C., Di Nardo, P.A., Rapee, R.M., & Barlow, D.H. (1990). Syndrome comorbidity in patients diagnosed with a DSM-III-R anxiety disorder. *Journal of Abnormal Psychology, 99,* 308–312.

Sanderson, W.C., & Wetzler, S. (1991). Chronic anxiety and generalized anxiety disorder: Issues in comorbidity. In R.M. Rapee & D.H. Barlow (Eds.), *Chronic anxiety: Generalized anxiety disorder and mixed anxiety-depression* (pp. 119–135). New York : Guilford Press.

Sanderson, W.C., Wetzler, S., Beck, A.T., & Betz, F. (1994). Prevalence of personality disorders among patients with anxiety disorders. *Psychiatry Research, 51,* 167–174.

Sareen, J., Cox, B.J., Clara, I., & Asmundson, G.J.G. (2005). The relationship between anxiety disorders and physical disorders in the U.S. National Comorbidity Survey. *Depression and Anxiety, 21,* 193–202.

Schneier, F.R., Heckelman, L.R., Garfinkel, R., Campeas, R., Fallon, B.A., Gitow, A., Street, L., Del Bene, D., Leibowitz, M.R. (1994). Functional impairment in social phobia. *Journal of Clinical Psychiatry, 55,* 322–331.

Schut, A., Pincus, A., Castonguay, L.G., Bedics, J., Kline, M., Long, D., & Seals, K. (1997,November). *Perceptions of attachment and self-representations at best and worst in generalized anxiety disorder.* Paper presented at the annual meeting of the Association for the Advancement of Behavior Therapy, Miami.

Scogin, F., Rickard, H.C., Keith, S., Wilson, J., & McElreath, L. (1992). Progressive and imaginal relaxation training for elderly persons with subjective anxiety. *Psychology and Aging, 7,* 419–424.

Segal, Z.V., Williams, J.M.G., & Teasdale, J.D. (2002). *Mindfulness-Based Cognitive Therapy for Depression: A new approach to preventing relapse.* New York: Guilford Press.

Sexton, K.A., & Dugas, M.J. (2008). The Cognitive Avoidance Questionnaire: Validation of the English translation. *Journal of Anxiety Disorders, 22,* 355–370.

Shafran, R., Thordarson, D.S., & Rachman, S. (1996). Thought-action fusion in obsessive compulsive disorder. *Journal of Anxiety Disorders, 10,* 379–391.

Sheehan, D.V. (1983). *The Anxiety Disease.* New York: Scribner.

Sheehan, D.V., & Lecrubier, Y. (2002). *MINI International Neuropsychiatric Interview for DSM-IV* (English Version 5.0.0). Tampa: University of South Florida.

Sheehan, D.V., Lecrubier, Y., Harnett-Sheehan, K., Janavs, J., Weiller, E., Bonara, L.I., Keskiner, A., Schinka, J., Knapp, E., Sheehan, M.F., & Dunbar, G.C. (1997). Reliability and validity of the MINI International Neuropsychiatric Interview (M.I.N.I.): According to the SCID-P. *European Psychiatry, 12,* 232–241.

Shoenberger, D., & Hazlett-Stevens, H. (in press). Interpersonal problems linked to panic disorder with agoraphobia. To appear in *Advances in Psychology Research Volume 50.* New York: Nova Science Publishers, Inc.

Sinha, S.S., Mohlman, J., & Gorman, J.M. (2004). Neurobiology. In R.G. Heimberg, C.L. Turk, & D.S. Mennin (Eds.), *Generalized anxiety disorder: Advances in research and practice* (pp. 187–216). New York: Guilford Press.

Sinoff, G., Ore, l., Zlotogorsky, D., & Tamir, A. (1999). Short anxiety screening test: A brief instrument for detecting anxiety in the elderly. *International Journal of Geriatric Psychiatry, 14,* 1062–1071.

Slade, T., & Andrews, G. (2001). DSM-IV and ICD-10 generalized anxiety disorder: Discrepant diagnoses and associated disability. *Social Psychiatry and Psychiatric Epidemiology, 36,* 45–51.

Spielberger, C.D., Gorsuch, R.L., Lushene, R., Vagg, P.R., & Jacobs, G.A. (1983). *Manual of the State-Trait Anxiety Inventory.* Palo Alto, CA: Consulting Psychologists Press.

Spitzer, R.L., Kroenke, K., & Williams, J.B. (1999). Validation and utility of a self-report version of PRIME-MD: The PHQ primary care study. Primary Care Evaluation of Mental Disorders. Patient Health Questionnaire. *Journal of the American Medical Association, 282,* 1737–1774.

Spitzer, R.L., Williams, J.B., Gibbon, M., & First, M. (1988). *Structured Clinical Interview for DSM-III-R-Patient Edition.* New York: Biomedical Research Department, New York State Psychiatric Institute.

Spitzer, R.L., Williams, J.B.W., Kroenke, K., Linzer, M., deGruy, F.V., Hahn, S.R., Brody, D., & Johnson, J.G. (1994). Utility of a new procedure for diagnosing mental disorders in primary care: The PRIME-MD 1000 study. *Journal of the American Medical Association, 272,* 1749–1756.

Stanley, M.A., Beck, J.G., & Glassco, J.D. (1996). Treatment of generalized anxiety in older adults: A preliminary comparison of cognitive-behavioral and supportive approaches. *Behavior Therapy, 27,* 565–581.

Stanley, M.A., Beck, J.G., Novy, D.M., Averill, P.M., Swann, A.C., Diefenbach, G.J., & Hopko, D.R. (2003). Cognitive-behavioral treatment of late-life generalized anxiety disorder. *Journal of Consulting and Clinical Psychology, 71,* 309–319.

Stanley, M.A., Beck, J.G., & Zebb, B. (1996). Psychometric properties of four anxiety measures in older adults. *Behaviour Research and Therapy, 34,* 827–838.

Stanley, M.A., Hopko, D.R., Diefenbach, G.J., Bourland, S.L., Rodriguez, H., & Wagener, P. (2003). Cognitive-behavior therapy for late-life generalized anxiety disorder in primary care: Preliminary findings. *American Journal of Geriatric Psychiatry, 11,* 92–96.

Stanley, M.A., & Novy, D.M. (2000). Cognitive behavior therapy for generalized anxiety disorder in late life. *Journal of Anxiety Disorders, 14,* 191–207.

Stanley, M.A., Novy, D.M., Bourland, S.L., Beck, J.G., & Averill, P.M. (2001). Assessing older adults with generalized anxiety: A replication and extension. *Behaviour Research & Therapy, 39,* 221–235.

Starcevic, V., & Bogojevic, G. (1999). The concept of generalized anxiety disorder: Between the too narrow and too wide diagnostic criteria. *Psychopathology, 32,* 5–11.

Stein, M.B., & Heimberg, R.G. (2004). Well-being and life satisfaction in generalized anxiety disorder: Comparison to major depressive disorder in a community sample. *Journal of Affective Disorders, 79,* 161–166.

Stöber, J. (1998).Worry, problem solving, and suppression of imagery: The role of concreteness. *Behaviour Research and Therapy, 36,* 751–756.

Stöber, J., & Bittencourt, J. (1998). Weekly assessment of worry: An adaptation of the Penn State Worry Questionnaire for monitoring changes during treatment. *Behaviour Research and Therapy, 36,* 645–656.

Stöber, J., Tepperwien, S., & Staak, M. (2000). Worrying leads to reduced concreteness of problem elaborations: Evidence for the avoidance theory of worry. *Anxiety, Stress, and Coping, 13,* 217–227.

Summerfeldt, L.J., Antony, M.M. (2002). Structured and semistructured diagnostic interviews. In M.M. Antony, D.H. Barlow (Eds.), *Handbook of assessment and treatment planning for psychological disorders* (pp. 3–37). New York: Guilford Press.

Tallis, F., Davey, G.C.L., & Bond, A. (1994). The Worry Domains Questionnaire. In G.C.L. Davey & F. Tallis (Eds.), *Worrying: Perspectives on theory, assessment, and treatment* (pp. 61–89). Chichester, UK: Wiley.

Tallis, F., Eysenck, M., & Matthews, A. (1992). A questionnaire for the measurement of nonpathological worry. *Personality and Individual Differences, 13,* 161–168.

Thayer, J.F., Friedman, B.H., & Borkovec, T.D. (1996). Autonomic characteristics of generalized anxiety disorder and worry. *Biological Psychiatry, 39,* 255–266.

Tollefson, G.D., Tollefson, S.L., Pederson, M., Luxenberg, M., & Dunsmore, G. (1991). Comorbid irritable bowel syndrome in patients with generalized anxiety and major depression. *Annals of Clinical Psychiatry, 3,* 215–222.

Turk, C.L., Heimberg, R.G., Luterek, J.A., Mennin, D.S., & Fresco, D.M. (2005). Emotion dysregulation in generalized anxiety disorder: A comparison with social anxiety disorder. *Cognitive Therapy and Research, 29,* 89–106.

Turk, C.L., Heimberg, R.G., & Mennin, D.S. (2004). Assessment. In R.G. Heimberg, C.L. Turk, & D.S. Mennin (Eds.), *Generalized anxiety disorder: Advances in research and practice* (pp. 219–247). New York: Guilford Press.

Van Rijsoort, S., Emmelkamp, P., & Vervaeke, G. (1999). The Penn State Worry Questionnaire and the Worry Domains Questionnaire: Structure, reliability, and validity. *Clinical Psychology and Psychotherapy, 6,* 297–307.

Vasey, M.W. & Borkovec, T.D. (1992). A catastrophizing assessment of worrisome thoughts. *Cognitive Therapy and Research, 16,* 1–16.

Vrana, S.R., Cuthbert, B.N., & Lang, P.J. (1986). Fear imagery and text processing. *Psychophysiology, 23,* 247–253.

Warda, G., & Bryant, R.A. (1998). Thought control strategies in acute stress disorder. *Behaviour Research and Therapy, 36,* 1171–1175.

Waters, A.M., & Craske, M.G. (2005). Generalized anxiety disorder. In M.M. Antony, D.R. Ledley, & R.G. Heimberg (Eds.), *Improving outcomes and preventing relapse in cognitive-behavioral therapy* (pp. 77–127). New York: Guilford.

Watson, D., Clark, L.A., Tellegen, A. (1988). Development and validation of brief measures of positive and negative affect: The PANAS scales. *Journal of Personality and Social Psychology, 54,* 1063–1070.

Watson, D., Weber, K., Assenheimer, J.S., Clark, L.A., Strauss, M.E., & McCormick, R.A. (1995). Testing a tripartite model: I. Evaluating the convergent and discriminant validity of anxiety and depression symptom scales. *Journal of Abnormal Psychology, 104,* 3–14.

Watts, A. (1975). *Tao: The watercourse way.* New York: Pantheon Books.

Wegner, D.M. (1989). *White bears and other unwanted thoughts: Suppression, obsession, and the psychology of mental control.* New York: The Guilford Press.

Wells, A. (1994). A multi-dimensional measure of worry: Development and preliminary evaluation of the Anxious Thoughts Inventory. *Anxiety, Stress, and Coping, 6,* 289–299.

Wells, A. (2000). *Emotional disorders and metacognition: Innovative cognitive therapy.* New York: John Wiley & Sons Ltd.

Wells, A. (2004). A cognitive model of GAD: Metacognitions and pathological worry. In R.G. Heimberg, C.L. Turk, & D.S. Mennin (Eds.), *Generalized anxiety disorder: Advances in research and practice* (pp. 3–28). New York: Guilford Press.

Wells, A. (2005). The Metacognitive Model of GAD: Assessment of Meta-Worry and Relationship with DSM-IV Generalized Anxiety Disorder. *Cognitive Therapy and Research, 29,* 107–121.

Wells, A., & Carter, K. (1999). Preliminary tests of a cognitive model of generalized anxiety disorder. *Behaviour Research and Therapy, 37,* 585–594.

Wells, A., & Carter, K. (2001). Further tests of a cognitive model of generalized anxiety disorder: Metacognitions and worry in GAD, panic disorder, social phobia, depression, and nonpatients. *Behavior Therapy, 32,* 85–102.

Wells, A., & Davies, M.I. (1994). The Thought Control Questionnaire: A measure of individual differences in the control of unwanted thoughts. *Behaviour Research and Therapy, 32,* 871–878.

Wells, A., & King, P. (2005). Metacognitive therapy for generalized anxiety disorder: An open trial. *Journal of Behavior Therapy and Experimental Psychiatry, 37,* 206–212.

Wells, A., & Papageorgiou, C. (1995). Worry and the incubation of intrusive images following stress. *Behaviour Research and Therapy, 33,* 579–583.

Wetherell, J.L., Gatz, M., Craske, M.G. (2003). Treatment of generalized anxiety disorder in older adults. *Journal of Consulting and Clinical Psychology, 71,* 31–40.

Wetherell, J.L., Hopko, D.R., Diefenbach, G.J., Averill, P.M., Beck, J.G., Craske, M.G., Gatz, M., Novy, D.M., & Stanley, M.A. (2005). Cognitive-behavioral therapy for late-life generalized anxiety disorder: Who gets better? *Behavior Therapy, 36,* 147–155.

White, J., Keenan, M., & Brooks, N. (1992). Stress control: A controlled comparative investigation of large group therapy for generalized anxiety disorder. *Behavioural Psychotherapy, 20,* 97–114.

Wisocki, P., Handen, B., & Morse, C. (1986). The Worry Scale as a measure of anxiety among homebound and community active elderly. *The Behavior Therapist, 5,* 91–95.

Wittchen, H., Zhao, S., Kessler, R.C., & Eaton, W.W. (1994). DSM-III-R generalized anxiety disorder in the National Comorbidity Survey. *Archives of General Psychiatry, 51,* 355–364.

Wolpe, J. (1958). *Psychotherapy by reciprocal inhibition.* Stanford: Stanford University Press.

Woodman, C.L., Noyes, R., Black, D.W., Schlosser, S., & Yagla, S.J. (1999). A 5-year follow-up study of generalized anxiety disorder and panic disorder. *Journal of Nervous and Mental Disease, 187,* 3–9.

World Health Organization. (1992). *International classification of diseases and related health problems* (10th ed.). Geneva: World Health Organization.

World Health Organization. (1997). *Composite International Diagnostic Interview, version 2.1.* Geneva: World Health Organization.

Yerkes, R.M., & Dodson, J.D. (1908). The relation of strength of stimulus to rapidity of habit-formation. *Journal of Comparative Neurology and Psychology, 18,* 459–482.

Yesavage, J.A., Sheikh, J.I., Tanke, E.D. & Hill, R. (1988). Response to memory training and individual differences in verbal intelligence and state anxiety. *American Journal of Psychiatry, 145,* 636–639.

Yonkers, K.A., Dyck, I.R., Warshaw, M., & Keller, M.B. (2000). Factors predicting the clinical course of generalized anxiety disorder. *British Journal of Psychiatry, 176,* 544–549.

Yonkers, K.A., Warshaw, M., Massion, A., & Keller, M.B. (1996). Phenomenology and course of generalized anxiety disorder. *British Journal of Psychiatry, 168,* 308–313.

Zanarini, M.C., Skodol, A.E., Bender, D., Dolan, R., Sanislow, C., Schaefer, E., Morey, L.C., Grilo, C.M., Shea, M.Y., McGashan, T.H., & Gunderson, J.G. (2000). The collaborative longitudinal personality disorder study: Reliability of Axis I and II diagnoses. *Journal of Personality Disorders, 14,* 291–299.

Zimmerman, M., & Mattia, J.I. (1999). The reliability and validity of a screening questionnaire for 13 DSM-IV Axis I disorders (the Psychiatric Diagnostic Screening Questionnaire) in psychiatric outpatients. *Journal of Clinical Psychiatry, 60,* 677–683.

Zimmerman, M., & Mattia, J.I. (2001a). The Psychiatric Diagnostic Screening Questionnaire: Development, reliability, and validity. *Comprehensive Psychiatry, 42,* 175–189.

Zimmerman, M., & Mattia, J.I. (2001b). A self-report scale to help make psychiatric diagnoses: The Psychiatric Diagnostic Screening Questionnaire (PDSQ). *Archives of General Psychiatry, 58,* 787–794.

Zinbarg, R.E., Craske, M.G., & Barlow, D.H. (2006). *Mastery of your anxiety and worry: Therapist guide* (2nd ed.). New York: Oxford University Press.

Zuellig, A.R., Newman, M.G., Kachin, K.E., & Constantino, M.J. (1997, November). *Differences in parental attachment profiles in adults diagnosed with generalized anxiety disorder, panic disorder, or non-disordered.* Paper presented at the 31st Annual Convention of the Association for Advancement of Behavior Therapy, Miami, FL.

# Index

.